DEALING WITH DEMENTIA FOR CAREGIVERS

DEALING WITH DEMENTIA FOR CAREGIVERS:

Real-World Advice to Prevent & Relieve Crisis Situations, Manage Long Care Hours, Alleviate the Burden You Feel & Cope with Daily Frustrations

***

S. R. Hatton

© Copyright 2024 - All rights reserved.

The content contained within this book may not be reproduced, duplicated, or transmitted without direct written permission from the author or the publisher.

Under no circumstances will any blame or legal responsibility be held against the publisher or author for any damages, reparation, or monetary loss due to the information contained within this book, either directly or indirectly.

Legal Notice:

This book is copyright-protected. It is only for personal use. You cannot amend, distribute, sell, use, quote, or paraphrase any part of the content within this book without the consent of the author or publisher. In addition, this book contains some content that has been generated using artificial intelligence (AI) technology, including some of the images, for the purpose of avoiding any plagiarism and/or copyright issues.

Disclaimer Notice:

Please note that the information contained within this document is for educational and entertainment purposes only. All efforts have been executed to present accurate, up-to-date, reliable, and complete information. No warranties of any kind are declared or implied. Readers acknowledge that the author is not engaged in the rendering of legal, financial, medical, or professional advice. The content within this book has been derived from various sources. Please consult a licensed professional before attempting any techniques outlined in this book.

By reading this document, the reader agrees that under no circumstances is the author responsible for any losses, direct or indirect, that are incurred as a result of the use of the information contained within this document, including, but not limited to, errors, omissions, or inaccuracies.

***

© 2024 by S. R. Hatton Publishing

All rights reserved. This book or any portion thereof may not be reproduced or used in any manner whatsoever without the author's express written permission except for the use of brief quotations in a book review.

Printed in the United States of America
First Printing, 2024
ISBN 979-8-9885202-0-7
Bottom Line Solutions, LLC
DBA S. R. Hatton Publishing
Contact email: SRHatton@bottomlinesolutions.net

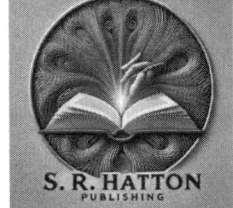

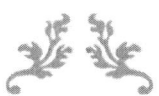

This book is dedicated to my Grandma Bonnie, a sweet soul—even when dementia had her completely within its grip—whose favorite saying was "Oh, happy day!" Her feisty spirit forever dwells in the hearts of those who were lucky enough to know her.

Prologue

My dearest readers and fellow caregivers, get ready to experience a reading revolution! I am thrilled to introduce a feature that merges the best of both worlds: traditional and digital reading. To ensure everyone can access the treasure trove of resources found within the hyperlinks of the digital version, I have embedded QR codes right into the paperback edition.

I know many of you love the feel of an actual book in your hands, flipping through pages and revisiting bookmarked sections. But let's face it, ebooks have their perks, too, like instant access to hyperlinks leading to web pages or PDFs brimming with crucial information. So, why should ebook readers have all the fun?

That's why I've plopped QR codes into my printed books alongside each digital hyperlink.* Now, anyone with a smartphone can scan these codes and be whisked away to extra content, enhancing your reading experience without leaving the page.

It's a simple yet genius way to elevate your reading journey, ensuring that everyone—no matter their format preference—gets the full scoop. This interactive twist modernizes the reading experience, bringing new levels of engagement and accessibility to each page.

Not sure how QR codes work? No worries! Let's do a test run. Grab your smartphone and open the camera. Now, hold it up as if you are about to snap a photo of the QR code below, but DON'T actually take the picture.

*Please note that I did not include a QR code for each hyperlink that corresponds with the 'References' at the end of the book—to avoid all the clutter that would cause.

vi | Prologue

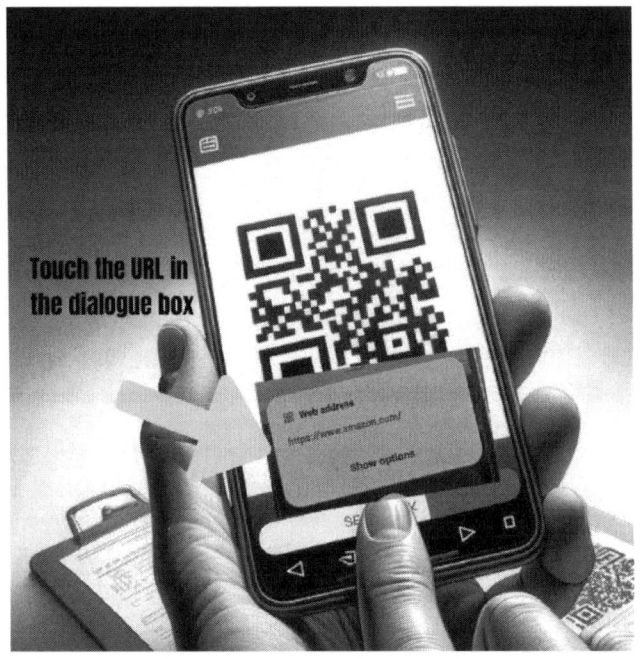

Now, touch the URL in the dialogue box that shows up on your camera screen (see above). And, Bam! You've just landed on Amazon.com via your smartphone! If now is not a good time to dive in and read the content, simply send it to yourself using whatever tech wizardry you prefer—email, text, carrier pigeon—and check it out later on your laptop or tablet. You're all set for a reading adventure that's as rich as a triple chocolate cake. Happy scanning!

For those of you rockin' the ebook version, you'll click hyperlinks that show up (like HERE), and you'll be whisked away to the same fabulous resource. Technology is like a magical unicorn, prancing around and sprinkling your life with convenience—if you know how to harness it! 🦄

Table of Contents

Prologue v
Introduction x
    The Journey Ahead xii
    What Are Your Expectations? xiii
    The Superhero's Guide to Dementia Caregiving xiii
    Summary of Chapters xiv

Chapter 1: Trapped in the Maze: Understanding the Complexity of Dementia 1
    The Unforgiving Sickness 1
    What Is Dementia? 3
        Alzheimer's Disease   5
        Frontotemporal Dementia (FTD)   7
        Lewy Body Dementia   9
        Vascular Dementia   12
        Mixed Dementia   14
    A Day in the Life of a Dementia Patient 15
    Can I Avoid Getting Dementia? 18
    Risk Factors Associated With Dementia 18
    Ways to Delay Dementia 20

Chapter 2: Diagnosing Dementia: Unraveling the Clues 22
    Opening Pandora's Box: Approaching the Subject of Dementia Diagnosis 22
    Persuading Your Loved One to Get Tested 23
    The Path to Dementia Diagnosis 24
    Financial and Legal Planning—The Earlier, the Better 26
    Bridging the Gap: Accessing Vital Support for Dementia Caregiving 28
    The Emotional Impact of a Dementia Diagnosis 29

Chapter 3: Real-World Advice for Major Caregiving Hurdles 32
    Heartbreak and Hallucinations 32
    To Pretend or Not to Pretend 33
    Shedding Some Light on Sundowning 34

    Supporting Your Loved One Through Sunset 36
    Sundowning Advice from Caregivers 38

Chapter 4: A Caregiver's Guide to the Galaxy 40

    Sweet Acceptance: Embracing Gratitude and Releasing Bitterness 40

    There's Always More to Learn.. 41

    Dancing Through Dialogue: Tips for Effective Communication........................42

    From Overwhelmed to Order: Strategies to Efficiently Manage Daily Tasks 46

        Creating a Personalized Checklist of Enjoyable Activities   47

        Activity Ideas to Include in Your Daily/Weekly Planner   48

    Exploring Unconventional Therapies for Your Loved One..................................50

        Reminiscence and Life Story Work   50

        Strategies for Success   53

        Essential Inclusions   53

    Guided by the Mind: A Revolutionary Dementia Therapy 54

    It's Not Just for Your LOWD 57

Chapter 5: There's No Place Like Home 62

    The Vulnerability of Dementia Sufferers in Their Own Backyard 62

    Building a Dementia-Friendly Home: Colors, Patterns, and Consistency 63

        Practical Home Tips   64

        The Art of Dementia-Friendly Flooring   65

        Easy Eating & Drinking Tips   66

        Bathroom Necessities   66

        Maintaining Continuity: Clear Labels & Familiar Objects   67

        Promoting Safety: A Protected Environment   68

        Minimizing Fall Risks   69

        Wandering—A Prevailing Risk & Some Precautions   69

Chapter 6: The Mid-Stage Maze.. 72

    Thriving Through the Challenges of Middle-Stage Dementia 72

    What to Anticipate in the Middle Stages.. 75

    Real-World Tips & Tricks for Middle-Stage Dementia 77

Chapter 7: What To Do When What You Do Just Isn't Enough 95

    Handling Hospital Hurdles: When Hospitalization Makes Sense 95

Comfort First: Introducing Palliative Care for Your LOWD 96
Recognizing When It's Time for Memory Care 98
    Finding the Right Memory Care Facility   99
    Preparing for the Transition   100
    Adjusting to the New Normal   100
    Ensuring Quality Care   100
    Navigating Healthcare Advocacy for Your Loved One   101
    Becoming the Voice: Advocacy in Medical Settings   101

Chapter 8: The Caregiver's Caretaker **104**
    The Invisible Second Patient—You 104
    Course Correction: Overcoming & Preventing Caregiving Mistakes 106
    Common Caregiving Mistakes & the Most Common Solutions 106
    Unchecked Stress: The Silent Saboteur in Caregiving 115
    Shaping Your Stress: From Chronic Burden to Healthy Catalyst 116
    What Is Caregiver Burnout? 118
        Burnout Quiz   119
    Real-World Tips & Tricks to Deal with Caregiver Burnout 122

Chapter 9: Handling the Inevitable with Grace **127**
    I Hate, I Hate, I Hate! 127
    The Expected Visitor 128
    Reaching the End of the Road with Dementia 129
    Real-World Advice on Facing Death 130

Conclusion **133**

Epilogue **135**
    References 138

Introduction

"Cherish every moment you spend with those you love, no matter how fleeting it may seem nor how heavy it weighs upon you." —S.R. Hatton

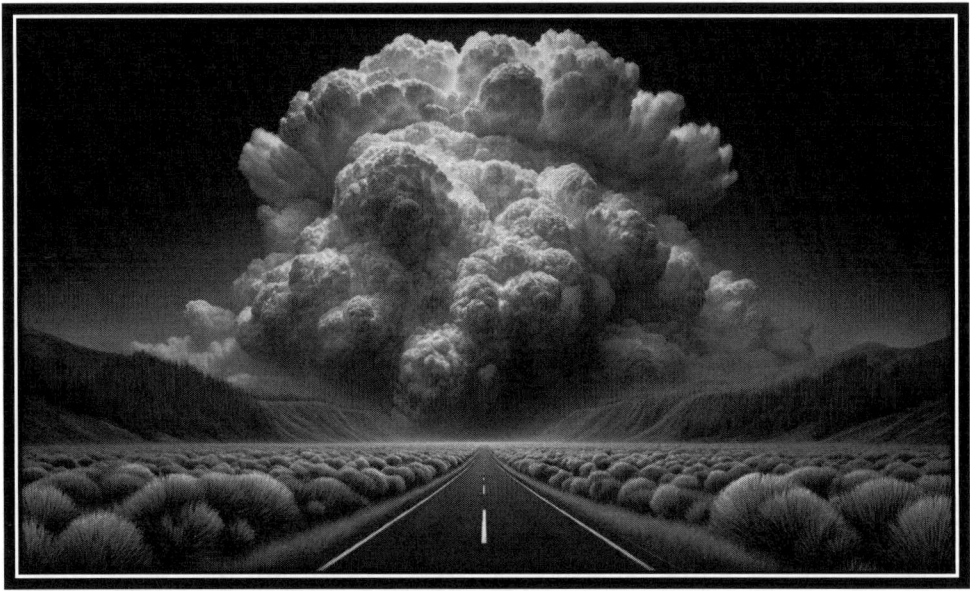

*"When I come to the end of the road
And the sun has set for me
I want no rites in a gloom-filled room
Why cry for a soul set free?
Miss me a little, but not for long
And not with your head bowed low
Remember the love that once we shared
Miss me, but let me go.
For this is a journey we all must take
And each must go alone.
It's all part of the master plan
A step on the road to home.
When you are lonely and sick at heart
Go to the friends you know.
Laugh at all the things we used to do
Miss me, but let me go."*

—Christina Rossetti, Let Me Go

By the time you finish reading this sentence—or about **every three seconds**—somewhere in the world, someone's life is dramatically changed by dementia. As of 2020, over 55 million people were already navigating this challenging journey, and projections suggest that by 2050, that number will skyrocket to 139 million (*ADI - Dementia Statistics*, n.d.). These aren't just dry statistics; they embody a vast, dynamic community of caregivers just like you, all rallying to brave the storm together.

In "Dealing with Dementia for Caregivers," I poured my heart, soul, and countless tears into creating a guide that's both deeply practical and genuinely supportive. This book is packed with an array of tips, tricks, and resources designed to help you manage crises, trim down long caregiving hours, alleviate burdens, and soothe your daily frustrations. Built on the latest research and innovative strategies, this guide is your ally, crafted to enhance your well-being and that of your loved one.

Hi, I'm Shanlynn. My own dance with dementia began many years ago with my beloved grandmother's diagnosis. But this cruel disease didn't stop there; it cast a shadow over my mother, her sister, and, it seems, even me. Although we haven't yet confirmed the presence of the dreaded APOE-e4 gene, I would bet the farm that it is lurking in our DNA.

My ordeal began unexpectedly in May 2020 with a flurry of unexplained, debilitating symptoms. After exhaustive testing and consultations that culminated in a disheartening encounter at Mayo Clinic, where the best advice was, "You'll just have to live with it," I was left grappling with more questions than answers. The discovery of unusual white matter hyperintensities in my brain hinted at the early onset of dementia—a prospect both terrifying and mystifying to me.

Driven by a need for clarity and understanding, I immersed myself deeply into the world of dementia. This book distills everything I've learned from extensive research, discussions in online forums, and countless hours spent digesting every available resource on dementia care. It is designed to arm you with knowledge, offering practical tips and heartfelt advice to navigate the complexities of caregiving.

But this isn't just an assembly of facts; it's a heartfelt conversation from one weary warrior to another. Consider this book your trusted sidekick—a friend who understands, listens, and supports you. As you turn these pages, you'll hear from countless caregivers who have transformed their daily chaos into moments of triumph.

These past few years have revealed a resilience I didn't know I had, and my greatest hope is that the stories and strategies in this book will ignite that same resilient spirit in you. Together, let's shine a light on even the darkest corners of dementia, empowering each other to face this journey with knowledge, support, and unwavering courage.

The Journey Ahead

Navigating the path with loved ones who have dementia is like being thrown into an emotional blender set to 'high.' Sure, the transformation is inevitable—emotional and physical demands that make you question reality when your loved one may not even recognize you. But instead of stressing over the 'what-ifs,' why not squeeze every last drop of wisdom from this book like it's a lemon and take it one chaotic moment at a time?

If you're still reading, you're probably yearning for a magical map to guide you to the 'end,' praying someone can shine a light on this shadowy journey. You already know it's a rollercoaster of epic proportions, draining you faster than your phone battery at 1%. When people chirp 'self-care,' you probably want to throw a pillow at them, screaming, "Who the hell has time for that?" But here's the kicker: Self-care isn't a luxury; it's your secret weapon. Ignoring it is like trying to juggle flaming swords—you're bound to get burned, and so will everyone around you.

Dementia can turn your loved one into a puzzle with missing pieces, bringing unpredictable waves of fear and confusion into your daily life. Remember, **these challenges are the disease talking, not your loved one**. (Yep, I know, this phrase is very over-used in the dementia caregiving arena, but it really is true.) But I've built this book to be your toolkit, packed with strategies to tackle these curveballs with resilience and maybe even a touch of grace.

Yes, the road is tough—and anyone who tries to convince you otherwise needs to be inducted into the Society of Bonkers. But my mission here is to enrich your caregiving journey, turning each step into a growth spurt of empathy and strength. The beauty of caregiving is that it molds you into a better human being—stronger, kinder, and more fulfilled.

The unpredictability of this path is daunting, but a little preparation can empower you. The changes you'll go through are profound, and this book offers practical advice to smooth your journey and boost your resilience. Remember, this path to 'the end' isn't a race—it's just another part of life's wild ride. So, buckle up, and let's get through it together.

What Are Your Expectations?

Look, I get it—talking about dementia caregiving is not exactly the stuff of feel-good bedtime stories. But, hey, I'm not about to let this book turn into a dreary slog through the swamp of sadness. We are all doing a frantic tango with Father Time, and we could use a chuckle or two to keep from stepping on our own toes. So brace yourself because these pages won't be your garden-variety guidebook droning on with the same old tips. If I can inject a little pep into your step for even half an hour, I'll pop the champagne and call it a win.

Now, picture yourself as the captain of a slightly wonky ship sailing the high seas of dementia care. Watching someone you love fade into the fog is nothing short of brutal. But here's the plot twist: amidst the storm, you're morphing into something mighty. This isn't just a journey through rough waters; it is an epic quest turning you into a caregiving superhero, complete with an arsenal of self-care magic and resilience.

And who knows? This gig might just steer you toward new horizons, career-wise. Think of it: all this hands-on caregiving experience could launch you into a bona fide profession. It's happening to folks everywhere, spinning an unexpected role into a calling filled with purpose. You're in the trenches, gaining insights and skills that are golden in the world of dementia care—a field that's crying out for heroes (literally, millions of them). So, why not make a cape out of that bath towel and dive into transforming both your future and the landscape of caregiving? Your journey could light the way for others and even redefine your life's work. At a minimum, you can turn this voyage into an adventure of growth and discovery.

The Superhero's Guide to Dementia Caregiving

Think of caregiving not just as a job you got roped into, but as your new superhero origin story. It's less about tackling tissues and pills and more about mastering the arcane skills of patience, resilience, and heartfelt compassion. Flipping through this book isn't just reading—it's treasure hunting. Wield it as your trusty sword, ready to slash through the murky mists of fear and caregiver chaos.

Within these pages lies a band of fellow superheroes—seasoned caregivers who have bared their souls, hoping you'll sidestep the traps they've already stumbled through. Sure, the road's got more twists than a pretzel factory, but with this compilation of know-how, you'll have everything you need to straighten things back up!

Summary of Chapters

Chapter 1: Dive into the wild world of neurological twists and turns where dementia stages get a full-blown exposé—from subtle brain blips to full-on cognitive fireworks. Grab strategies to ride this rollercoaster with the heart of a lion and the finesse of a seasoned pilot. (Quick sidenote here: Since the word 'cognitive' is going to be used quite often throughout this book, I want to define it right off the bat to avoid any confusion. In simple terms, the Collins Dictionary defines *cognitive* as "relating to the mental process involved in knowing, learning, and understanding things.")

Chapter 2: Strap in for a crash course in handling the "you've got dementia" bombshell without blowing a fuse. This chapter isn't just about surviving the news—it's about thriving through it! Learn ninja-level coping strategies, dive into the murky waters of financial and legal planning, and discover where to fish for aid when you feel like you're drowning in paperwork and emotions. It's like a handy guide for the sanity-challenged.

Chapter 3: We're going deep into the heart-tugging world of "pre-goodbyes" for when your loved one is still here but kinda isn't. And as the sun dips low, so might your spirits with the twilight terrors of sundowning. Fear not! You'll get the inside scoop on mastering these nightly nuisances and keeping your cool when the evening antics kick in. It's like a survival kit for the haunted hours!

Chapter 4: Feeling a bit bitter about your unplanned role as a caregiver? We'll spin that frustration into finesse as you master the art of patience and understanding, turning every challenging day into a chance to strengthen your caregiving superpowers. You'll also find out how to talk the talk in Dementia-ese—decoding gibberish and directing daily do's and don'ts. (I've also slipped a juicy nugget into this chapter about a lesser-known therapy that could be a true game-changer for you and your loved one with dementia.)

Chapter 5: Turn your home into a dementia-friendly fortress where safety meets snug. Learn how to banish booby traps and create a cozy corner for calm.

Chapter 6: Ever wondered what the world looks like from inside the mind of someone with dementia? Sure, we've got the brain scans and doctor's notes, but only a real-time narration from a brain on a dementia tour could truly clue us in. Get comfy for this chapter, where you'll get the inside scoop on what it feels like to navigate the marathon middle stage of the disease.

Chapter 7: Welcome to the tightrope walk of deciding when to hospitalize your dementia-afflicted loved one—balancing those pesky medical must-dos with the "Wait, is this actually helping?" doubts. Dive into the world of early palliative care and decipher the hieroglyphics of medical advocating, all to ensure your decisions are as well-informed as they are heartfelt.

Chapter 8: Feeling like a squeezed-out sponge? This chapter serves up a cocktail of rejuvenation recipes to transform caregiver fatigue into fortified enthusiasm—with an optional burnout quiz to give you an inkling of just how stressed out you've become. (And **don't miss this**: Here is where you'll also find 62 of the most common caregiving mistakes and their most common solutions.)

Chapter 9: The final curtain call is never easy. Prepare for the heart-tugging farewell with grace and guts. This chapter holds your hand through the dance of departure, ensuring you both find peace.

Chapter 1: Trapped in the Maze: Understanding the Complexity of Dementia

"The heart always remembers the feeling of love and being loved, even if the mind forgets." –S.R. Hatton

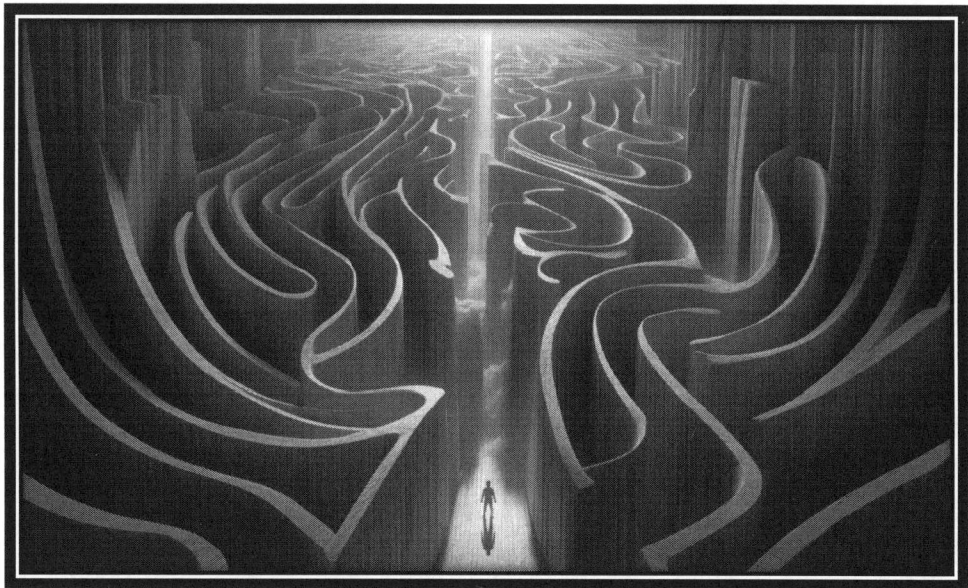

The Unforgiving Sickness

Trying to navigate dementia is like trying to solve a Rubik's Cube that changes its own stickers. One minute, your loved one with dementia (let's call them your "LOWD" to save some trees) is as clear as a sunny day, and the next, they're in a whirlpool of confusion, making the floor feel as stable as a unicycle on a tightrope. Their unexpected outbursts? They're like plot twists in a surreal novel where you're the bewildered protagonist who's accidentally wandered into the wrong story.

And if you're the type who tries to handle everything in caregiving land by being reasonable, rational, and logical, then STOP—because you're doing it wrong! Instead, think of yourself as a tourist in their delusional, topsy-turvy town. As the dementia disco progresses, you'll feel more like you accidentally gate-crashed their mental party. While it may seem like their brain has put up a 'Do Not Disturb' sign, trust me, they still need you—because it's not your gray matter staging a rebellion.

If you're setting up camp in the land of 'Normal,' you might want to pack up. In Dementia World, 'normal' is as reliable as a chocolate teapot. It's like trying to catch a cloud—pointless and frustrating. Dementia doesn't play fair; it's the game master of a board game with ever-changing rules.

Being a dementia caregiver is like riding a rollercoaster that only goes up in emotional intensity. Your LOWD might start seeing you as the villain in their personal epic, utterly oblivious to the capes you change into each and every day. Although playing the hero in this saga often feels like a thankless quest, armed with patience, understanding, and a knack for improvisation, you'll make this journey smoother for both of you.

The more you dive into the world of dementia, the more your empathy muscles bulk up. Let their bizarro reality steer your ship. If they declare it's snowing in July, just roll with it—build an imaginary snowman instead of correcting them. Arguing is about as effective as trying to teach a cat how to text.

Sure, dementia is a beast, but don't let it cloud your view of the person you cherish, who's now being kind of held hostage by their own brain. Remember, they are still the superstar you adore, not just the lead character in this twisty drama. Dementia might be snatching pieces of them away bit by bit, but your mission, which I assume you've already chosen to accept, is to deliver top-notch care.

This guidebook isn't just a flashlight in the murky waters of dementia—it is your submarine. From Chapter 3 on, we'll dive deeper into understanding this beast, its antics, and how to be the best darn caregiver you can be. Armed with knowledge, you'll navigate these choppy waters like the captain of the cheer squad—full of heart, courage, and ready to cheer on your LOWD, come rain or shine.

[Handwritten note: Loved One with dementia]

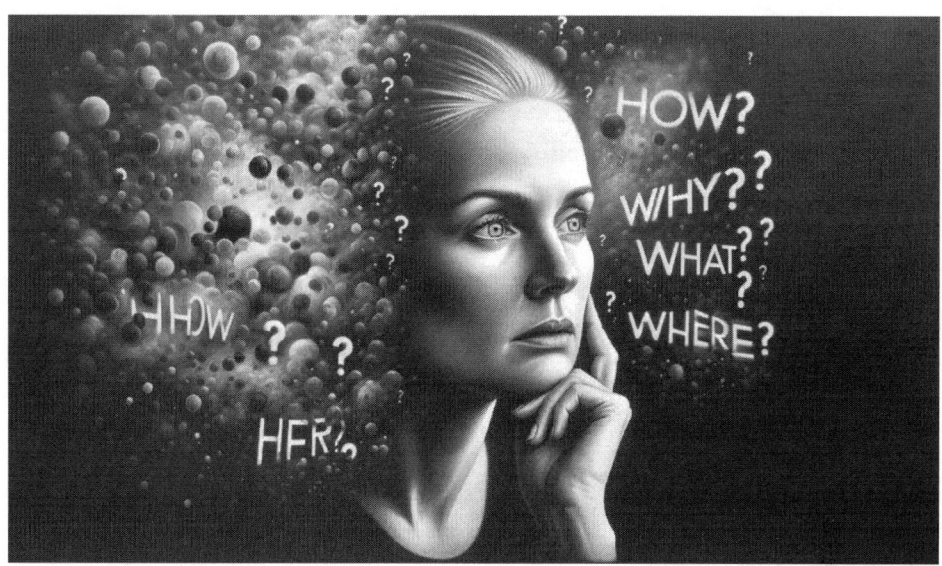

What Is Dementia?

To really understand your LOWD's condition—and the downward spiral that happens to them, you need a better understanding of what dementia actually **is**. At its most basic level, dementia isn't even a disease; it's a general term for the impaired ability to remember, think, or make decisions—which interferes with doing everyday activities (*What Is Dementia? | CDC*, n.d.).

Whether you're already certain your loved one has some form of dementia, or you've purchased this book looking for a little confirmation that you're right, take a look at this list of the most common behaviors that point toward a looming dementia diagnosis (remember, signs and symptoms can vary depending on the type and stage):

> **Memory Mayhem:** Forgets where they parked the car in their own driveway.
> **Word Soup:** Struggles to chat or read, turning dinner conversation into a game of charades.
> **Lost & Not Found:** Wanders off in the neighborhood, searching for their house... while standing in front of it.
> **Fiscal Fumbles:** Handles money like a Monopoly game, trying to pay actual bills with hotel money.
> **Question Encore:** Asks "What's for dinner?" so often it feels like an echo in the Grand Canyon.
> **Creative Naming:** Calls a watch a wrist clock because... well, it makes sense.
> **Slow-Mo Mode:** Takes an hour to make a sandwich, turning lunch prep into a slow-motion movie scene.

- **Interest Blackout:** Loses interest in watching football (or any favorite thing), even with front-row seats from the couch.
- **Imaginary Friends & Foes:** Has conversations with long-gone Uncle Pete and argues with invisible intruders.
- **Impulse Shopping:** Buys 20 cans of beans on impulse because, suddenly, they're prepping for an apocalypse.
- **Empathy Evasion:** Laughs during sad movies, missing the emotional cues.
- **Balance Boogie:** Tries a new dance move every time they stand up, wobbling like a toddler on ice skates. (*What Is Dementia? Symptoms, Types, and Diagnosis*, 2022)

Basically, dementia is like a shadowy specter that haunts the mind, slowly obscuring clarity, altering feelings, distorting behaviors, and reshaping the perception of reality. The culprit? Neurological diseases and other medical conditions, waging a stealthy campaign against the brain's ability to function at full capacity. It's a slow, creeping siege that gnaws at the crucial cognitive abilities needed for daily life.

Imagine the brain as a vibrant city, buzzing with activity. Dementia is akin to a silent, relentless blackout that engulfs the city, leaving its residents, or in this case, the individual, estranged from their sense of self. As the dementia worsens, memories fade into oblivion, and their former identity becomes a distant echo.

In your role as a caregiver, it's imperative to remember that your LOWD is more than just their medical condition. Think of their brain as a complex computer system, where dementia is like a malicious virus wreaking havoc on the hard drive. This hard drive—the hippocampus, the memory storage unit of the brain—is under constant assault, leading to erratic or non-functioning recall. Sometimes, they might encounter a system freeze; other times, they're faced with the equivalent of a 'blue screen of death,' where your presence in their memory is lost.

However, amidst this somber landscape, rays of hope persist. While dementia remains incurable as of now, various treatments can help manage symptoms and enhance the quality of life for individuals living with this condition. In some instances, these treatments can mitigate the damage and alleviate symptoms to a degree that allows for a more peaceful existence than one might anticipate.

In this chapter, we will navigate this maze of dementia—discussing the major neurological diseases such as Alzheimer's disease, Frontotemporal dementia (FTD), Lewy Body dementia (LBD), Vascular dementia, and Mixed dementia—all primary architects of this condition. I believe it's essential to understand these prevalent and potent instigators of dementia today. By expanding your knowledge, you will be better equipped to support your LOWD. And this, dear reader, is why it's absolutely vital for you to learn about it.

Alzheimer's Disease

Imagine Alzheimer's disease as an insidious architect, silently and relentlessly erecting serpentine structures of certain proteins—amyloid and tau—within the brain. With over 60 percent of dementia cases worldwide attributed to it, this prolific and unforgiving designer meticulously constructs barriers within the cerebral cortex. This process, a form of biochemical vandalism, shatters the lives of brain cells, leading to eroded thinking and a slow evaporation of memories. Age is its ally, with those over 60 finding themselves in its crosshairs, with the chances of an Alzheimer's diagnosis rising as the years pass by.

Envision the scale of this disease, knowing it can take a decade or two for these protein structures to cause enough damage to the brain cells. Once they infiltrate beyond the cerebral cortex, the affected individuals find the fortress of their self-sufficiency breached, rendering them unable to function independently.

Former American President Ronald Reagan was one notable figure who brought his battle into the public spotlight. In a poignant revelation made in November 1994, Reagan shared his personal struggle with Alzheimer's disease, an adversary as unforgiving as any he'd faced in his political career. His fight against this formidable foe lasted over a decade, ending at the age of 93 when he succumbed to pneumonia, a common but deadly complication of Alzheimer's (*Five things we learned from Reagan's Alzheimer's*, 2016).

In the U.S., research suggests a disproportionate impact of Alzheimer's on non-white demographics, with African Americans reported to be twice as susceptible as their white counterparts. Certain medical conditions, like the silent assassins diabetes and high blood pressure, stealthily elevate the risks of Alzheimer's in older individuals. If you're above 65, you're in the risk group for Alzheimer's, though remember, it isn't a certain fate (Right at Home, n.d.).

This knowledge is crucial because understanding the enemy is the first step to formulating a robust defense. Let this awareness ignite a desire for more learning and proactive steps in your journey of dealing with Alzheimer's, either personally or as a caregiver.

The Stages of Alzheimer's Disease

Stage 1: The Invisible Intruder

In the silent onset of Alzheimer's, the disease whispers its arrival, eluding detection while subtly infiltrating the brain. Just as a seed planted today does not blossom overnight, the trajectory from a healthy brain to full-blown Alzheimer's can span ten to twenty years. Early symptoms, most often cognitive impairments, can be so faint that they slip under the radar.

Stage 2: The Tug of Forgetfulness

Ever found yourself wandering aimlessly in a parking lot, searching for your car? Such episodes of forgetfulness are common and, in the hustle and bustle of life, not necessarily a harbinger of Alzheimer's. Yet, a marked increase in these moments, especially forgetting names, can be the disease gently tugging at your memory, signaling its presence. If this rings a bell, early intervention could help to decelerate Alzheimer's relentless march.

Stage 3: The Echoes of Memory Difficulties

When someone starts forgetting things more often, and it messes up their daily life, it's like their smooth day-to-day song is turning into a noisy mess. This might mean they're having trouble remembering things they've read, planning out their day, or even making their words fit together right. When things that used to be easy, like work or hanging out with friends, start to get tough, family and friends might notice that something's off. This is when it's really important to talk to a doctor who can help figure out what's going on and what to do next.

Stage 4: Recognizing the Later Stages of Alzheimer's

In the later stages of Alzheimer's disease, things get really tricky. The disease starts to mix up how a person uses words, figures out math, and organizes their day. This tough time can last for years. People might remember things from long ago better than what happened today. They could mix up what day it is, feel extra fidgety at night, act differently than they used to, feel more worried, or even see or believe things that aren't real. As everything around them starts to seem strange and unfamiliar, they might not feel like doing the activities they used to enjoy.

Stage 5: The Erosion of Independence

Here, the once-familiar landscape of daily life begins to crumble. Although still able to function, the affected individual may no longer manage solo living, forgetting those close to them and struggling with basic tasks like dressing.

Shadows of hallucinations, delusional behavior, and paranoia may start to creep in, slowly painting a surreal picture of their reality.

Stage 6: The Rise of Dependence

As Alzheimer's advances further, the patient begins to rely more heavily on others. Communication becomes a steep hill to climb, personality changes surface more frequently, and feelings of anxiety may swell. The dark clouds of hallucinations, paranoia, and delusions become more pronounced, often leading to fear and aggression. Now more than ever, medical intervention is critical to mitigate these severe symptoms.

Stage 7: The Seizure of Control

In the final stage, Alzheimer's assumes full control, hijacking both physical and mental capabilities. Like puppeteers pulling the strings, the disease dictates the person's ability to walk, eat, and even sit, necessitating round-the-clock supervision. As their immunity also takes a hit, they become more susceptible to infections. Ensuring their physical health, hygiene, and immunizations during this stage is crucial (Penn Medicine, 2020).

Frontotemporal Dementia (FTD)

Frontotemporal Dementia (FTD), an elusive shadow in the realm of neurological diseases, is diagnosed in only one in 20 dementia cases worldwide, making it a rarity among dementia types. This menacing intruder typically strikes early, asserting its presence between the ages of 45 to 65. The frontal and temporal lobes of the brain, like battlegrounds scarred by war, shrink due to the onslaught of cell damage, impairing language, movement, and speech. A sinister buildup of proteins in these areas is a hallmark of FTD, wreaking havoc on mood, emotional control, and the ability to plan.

Hollywood heart-stopper Bruce Willis is one of the latest notable figures to wrestle with this diagnosis. At the age of 67, the star previously grappled with aphasia—an ailment tarnishing the luster of effective communication—and found himself in the chilling embrace of FTD. The echoes of Willis' impaired speech and faltering interactions struck an eerie chord with his family, leaving them steeped in a whirlpool of shock, grief, and sadness.

His wife, Emma Heming Willis, has been seen navigating tidal waves of emotions, her eyes swollen with tears as she mourns the ebbing vitality of her husband's mind.

FTD is a relentless intruder, not unlike Alzheimer's, showing no mercy as it advances. Particularly among those under 60, it is a relatively common form of dementia-related illness. The disease, while incurable, can be managed with

ent, offering some respite from its onslaught. One of the more troubling facets of FTD is the erosion of empathy, a consequence of the disease's assault on emotional regulation.

As FTD progresses, its range of symptoms broadens, increasingly resembling Alzheimer's through its effects on memory loss. Everyday tasks, such as eating and swallowing, morph into Herculean challenges. Movement, once taken for granted, becomes a daunting hurdle, often necessitating assistance. The disease also leaves its mark on the patient's defenses, making them more susceptible to infections. Despite the grim reality, understanding and acknowledging the disease's progression can be a critical beacon guiding the path of care and support for those afflicted (Andrews, 2023).

The Stages of FTD

Stage 1: Subtle Cognitive Whispers

The initial stage of Frontotemporal Dementia might be as gentle as a whisper, with symptoms so mild they often escape notice. It's common to downplay early inconsistencies in a person's speech or mild antisocial tendencies as trivial. Subtle mood swings and dwindling empathy may provide the initial clues. Though faint, these signs begin to sketch the silhouette of FTD's arrival. Affected individuals may experience slight difficulties in articulating sentences or conveying thoughts and feelings. In this stage, the disease's footprints are faint, and life continues largely unaltered.

Stage 2: The Creeping Shadow of Change

As FTD progresses into its second stage, its impact becomes more pronounced. While symptoms are still not severe, there are clear changes in behavior that signal the disease's advancement. Individuals may exhibit increased forgetfulness, struggle more frequently with finding the right words, and begin neglecting daily tasks. These symptoms may stand out to friends and family, who might also see a noticeable decline in the person's sharpness of thought and clarity of speech.

Stage 3: The Battle with Language

In its third stage, FTD's progression quickens, turning mild symptoms into persistent and stark difficulties. Speech and language increasingly become significant barriers to communication. Memory loss deepens, and atypical behaviors occur more often. Social interactions may deteriorate into patterns that are not only unrecognizable but also potentially startling. Professional life is likely to suffer dramatically as difficulties in speaking create substantial obstacles to effective communication.

Stage 4: The Siege on Quality of Life

By the fourth stage of FTD, the symptoms significantly impair the individual's quality of life. Language difficulties become more severe, complicating everyday interactions. Individuals may find themselves unable to recall simple words during conversation, and other signs of dementia, such as severe memory loss and unpredictable behavior, become more evident. Additionally, a diminished sense of spatial orientation may cause confusion and disorientation in new surroundings, making it essential for them to receive assistance when moving around.

Stage 5: A Shift in Personality and Mood

In stage five, the quality of life continues to deteriorate significantly, with symptoms akin to those seen in advanced Alzheimer's disease becoming more pronounced each day. Cognitive functions decline sharply, and language and memory impairments deepen, severely hindering the ability to make decisions or manage self-care. At this point, patients typically require constant supervision to ensure their safety and prevent them from wandering or becoming lost. Additionally, physical rigidity may increase, making mobility a major challenge.

Stage 6: Memory's Retreat

As FTD advances into stage six, a retreat in speech, cognitive abilities, and memory echoes Alzheimer's typical patterns. Patients may become more isolated, signaling a decline in mental health. Falls and accidents become more frequent and dangerous, recovery from injuries harder, possibly confining patients to wheelchairs. The need for constant, hands-on care escalates dramatically.

Stage 7: The Final Curtain of Cognitive Decline

Stage seven marks FTD's final, most severe phase. Living alone becomes an impossibility as mental health and cognitive abilities spiral downward and all other symptoms worsen. Constant care becomes paramount as mobility challenges, speech issues, memory loss, and declining mental health present daily hurdles. This advanced stage of FTD makes patients vulnerable to infections and other illnesses, with conditions like pneumonia often proving fatal (Dementech, 2023).

Lewy Body Dementia

Lewy Body Dementia (LBD), as Susan Schneider, the widow of beloved actor Robin Williams, aptly named it, is a "terrorist inside the brain." Over a million lives in the United States are haunted by this insidious disease, often misdiagnosed as Parkinson's due to its uncanny resemblance in symptomology. Initial signs include movement challenges like shuffling walks, tremors, and muscular rigidity—symptoms common to Parkinson's as well. The villain in this tale, a Lewy Body, is a malevolent clump of protein that deposits itself across the brain's expanse.

Sharing the same relentless progression as Alzheimer's, LBD unfolds into a terrifying tableau of vivid hallucinations, delusions, and subtle memory slips. It gnaws at a person's mental capacity, crippling their ability to conduct daily tasks. It morphs peaceful sleep into a twisted circus filled with violent movements, unexpected falls from bed, and other bizarre behaviors. By interfering with the autonomous nervous system, it ushers in digestive troubles, heart palpitations, excessive sweating, and heightened blood pressure.

In the tragic case of Robin Williams, this silent adversary wasn't unmasked until after his passing, revealed only by a postmortem examination. Known for his battles with alcoholism and depression, the true enemy—LBD—hid in the shadows, leading to misdiagnoses and treatments aimed at depression. From 2013 to 2014, while on the set of *The Crazy Ones*, subtle hints of his struggle became evident: Robin would sometimes forget his lines, stumble, and fumble. As his disease worsened, nights became battlegrounds of unsettling delusions and tumultuous sleep. Once a social butterfly, he began to retract, his anxiety taking over.

In the months preceding his death, he grappled with a hallucination that one of his close friends was in grave danger. Despite reassurances and reality checks, Robin's mind was held hostage by this unfounded fear. He was being treated for Parkinson's disease and depression, not the true culprit—LBD. This undiagnosed brain damage, Schneider believes, was what tragically led Robin to suicide. Contrary to early media speculations, it wasn't depression or financial difficulties that ended his life; it was a battle against an unseen enemy within his brain (USA Today, 2020).

Stages of Lewy Body Dementia

Stage 1: The Quiet Before the Storm

In the initial stage of Lewy Body Dementia, it's all calm and quiet. No symptoms, no signs, no discernible changes—LBD remains a clandestine invader, yet to make its presence known.

Stage 2: A Ripple in the Pond

The tranquil surface of normalcy starts to ripple in the second stage. Though mild, the first signs appear as slight difficulties in communication—the struggle to find the perfect words to express feelings and thoughts. However, memory remains untouched, and the hustle and bustle of everyday life continue uninterrupted.

Stage 3: Beneath the Surface

As LBD evolves, the third stage brings a sea of change that's hard to overlook. Behaviors subtly shift, memory begins to falter, and managing finances turns into a challenging task.

Stage 4: The Onset of Mild Dementia

LBD pulls its victims deeper into its vortex in the fourth stage. Here, mild dementia sets in, erasing things like dates, names, and appointments from memory's slate. Tasks that were once routine now become hurdles in the day-to-day race.

Stage 5: From Moderate to Severe Dementia

As LBD advances to stage five, it turns crueler, wiping loved ones' names and familiar faces from memory. Everyday tasks turn into complex puzzles. The disease paints over personalities, ushering in mood swings and repetitious thoughts. New trials, like bladder issues, join the fray.

Stage 6: Deep into the Abyss of Decline

Diving deeper into the abyss of dementia, stage six sees the mind's tapestry unraveling at an alarming rate. Memory lapses become a constant companion. Everyday self-care deteriorates to a point where the comforting presence of a home-care companion becomes a necessity. Eating habits turn bizarre, and mood swings intensify. Delusions and hallucinations start their haunting dance, while speech falters and stumbles.

Stage 7: The Unraveling of the Self

In its final assault, LBD renders its victims bedridden, trapped in the twilight zone of their minds, and in dire need of round-the-clock care. Heartbreakingly, familiar faces blur into unrecognizable figures, and life's cherished memories dissolve into oblivion. The ability to communicate dwindles, and even eating becomes an extremely difficult task. In this advanced stage, control over bodily functions like bladder and bowel control tragically slips away (*7 Stages of Lewy Body Dementia*, n.d.).

Vascular Dementia

The iconic Iron Lady of Britain, former Prime Minister Margaret Thatcher, found herself ensnared in the merciless grip of vascular dementia after surviving a succession of mini-strokes. For a grueling stretch of 12 years, she valiantly waged war against dementia before surrendering to another stroke in April 2013, at the venerable age of 87. Stirred into action by their personal ordeal, the Thatcher family threw themselves into the mission of spreading awareness about the unseen enemy—dementia. Carol Thatcher, her daughter, penned a book encompassing their family's journey, poignantly illustrating how dementia cast a long shadow over her mother's later years. It came to a point where she had to constantly remind her mother of her father's passing, a fact Margaret would repeatedly forget (Learner, 2023).

Vascular dementia, a silent thief of cognitive abilities, is an aftermath of inadequate blood supply to the brain, often a grim consequence of a stroke. As was the case with Margaret Thatcher, her numerous mini-strokes over the years set the stage for the onset of vascular dementia. Strokes wage a war of attrition on the brain, laying waste to the blood vessels and choking off the life-sustaining oxygen supply to the brain. The resultant brain damage manifests as a haunting triad of memory loss, confusion, and concentration difficulties. Only falling second to Alzheimer's in its prevalence, vascular dementia is a formidable foe. Here's a glimpse into the challenging terrain of vascular dementia symptoms:

- A relentless march towards cognitive decline.
- An eroding ability to form sound judgments.
- Communication turns into a maze of obstacles.
- The secure fortress of memory begins to crumble.
- Physical challenges emerge, including swallowing difficulties and incontinence.
- Mobility turns into a taxing endeavor due to brain damage and oxygen deprivation.

Stages of Vascular Dementia

Stage 1: The Unseen Beginnings

Vascular dementia initially begins as a phantom. Silent, imperceptible changes take place in the brain due to oxygen deprivation, setting the stage for a long-drawn narrative that unfolds over the years, with no outward signs to hint at the unfolding story.

Stage 2: The Emergence of Subtle Confusion

A slight haze of confusion begins to cloud the mind of the patient, heralding a gentle dip in their cognitive abilities. Easily dismissed or overlooked, these early symptoms maintain their disguise, not quite raising any flags of concern yet.

Stage 3: The Arrival of Forgetfulness

As the tale progresses to the third stage, forgetfulness starts to weave its way into the narrative, albeit not at a rate that rings alarm bells. This gradual shift can extend over many years, subtly eroding the familiar contours of your loved one's persona before the change becomes palpable.

Stage 4: The Onset of Noticeable Cognitive Decline

Stage 4 announces itself as a clear turning point where dementia sheds its cloak of subtlety. Forgetfulness intensifies, tripping up the patient in their everyday tasks. From missing bill payments to losing track of recent meals, stage four lays down a trail of clues over several years.

Stage 5: The Advance Toward More Profound Cognitive Decline

Navigating life becomes a daunting challenge as the journey enters the more treacherous terrain of stage 5. Patients grapple with an escalating scale of forgetfulness, forgetting elementary tasks or vital details such as their address or phone number. Memories start playing tricks, with distant childhood recollections holding stronger than recent ones. The need for supervision and assistance becomes essential to see them through their daily routines.

Stage 6: The Threshold of Severe Cognitive Decline

The sixth stage pulls the rug from under the patient's feet, making independent living an unattainable dream. Unpleasant symptoms like incontinence emerge alongside difficulties in eating, while bouts of confusion intersperse their dwindling moments of clarity. Emotional turmoil often surfaces as aggression and anger.

Stage 7: The Endgame of Severe Cognitive Decline

In the final stage of this exhausting journey, most patients succumb to the relentless onslaught of vascular dementia. Completely reliant on round-the-clock care, they may be confined to their beds, stripped of their ability to engage with the world independently or articulate their thoughts (Dementech, 2022).

Mixed Dementia

The twilight years, beyond the age of 75, often cast an intricate shadow of mixed dementia on a significant number of individuals. This multifaceted condition typically weaves together threads of Alzheimer's disease and vascular dementia, although a variant that intertwines Lewy Body Dementia with Alzheimer's also makes its presence known. The journey through mixed dementia can oscillate wildly from person to person, depending heavily on the specific regions of the brain that are under siege. Often, it charges headlong into the more advanced stages of dementia, wielding a far heavier impact than any singular form of the disease.

A Duo of Decay: Alzheimer's and Vascular Dementia

This tag team represents the most frequent encounter in the world of mixed dementia. As two relentless diseases converge, they rapidly escalate the deterioration of the patient's condition, making the treatment a delicate dance of medical expertise. The person caught in this whirlwind bears the brunt of symptoms from both disorders, exposing them to a heightened vulnerability to other health complications.

A Lesser-Known Alliance: Lewy Body Dementia and Alzheimer's Disease

While less commonly encountered than its counterpart, the amalgamation of LBD and Alzheimer's is not an outlier in the spectrum of mixed dementia. This unique fusion imparts features absent in other types of dementia. It launches a concentrated assault on diverse brain regions, leading to a profound impairment in motor skills. Additionally, cognitive abilities, crucial for processing sensory information, crumble under its influence, spiraling the patient into a vortex of disorientation and confusion.

Stages of Mixed Dementia

Stage 1: The Calm Before the Storm

In the silent prologue of mixed dementia, no clear-cut signs emerge to signal the lurking presence of the disease. At this opening chapter, individuals still navigate their lives with their capabilities and independence intact.

Stage 2: The Faintest Whisper

The disease softly tiptoes into the second stage, where symptoms remain so gentle they're often dismissed as the harmless echoes of aging. Forgetfulness sprinkles mildly into their day, easily overlooked.

Stage 3: The Quiet Stirring

The third stage unfolds a modest tableau of symptoms, though none are alarming enough to trigger serious concern. The person, though grappling with forgetfulness, repetition, some memory loss, and occasional confusion, continues to hold the reins of their life.

Stage 4: The Rising Murmur

The waters start to churn in the fourth stage, with everyday tasks becoming daunting challenges. Carrying out everyday household chores, from cooking to doing laundry, or even making a phone call, can become overwhelmingly complex and challenging. Symptoms like incontinence, increasing forgetfulness, memory loss, numerical struggles, and social withdrawal start painting a more vivid picture of the disease.

Stage 5: The Unignorable Echoes

The fifth stage transforms the murmur into a persistent echo, as individuals start requiring aid to sail through the currents of daily tasks. The disease blurs the boundaries of locations and events, deepens memory loss, and renders personal details, like addresses or phone numbers, elusive. Even getting dressed transforms into a task necessitating an extra hand.

Stage 6: The Roaring Current

Stage six pours in like a tumultuous current, demanding comprehensive assistance for even the simplest tasks. Alongside the inability to use the bathroom or dress independently, patients may wander aimlessly, grapple with sleep disturbances, and fail to recall the names of loved ones. Familiar faces, though, still offer a thread of recognition amidst the storm.

Stage 7: The Thunderous Deluge

The finale of mixed dementia is a torrent of severity. In this concluding chapter, patients grapple with speech, lose awareness of their surroundings, require assistance during meals, and lose control over urination. Their muscular coordination routinely falters, rendering smiles, swallowing food, walking, or sitting upright a Herculean task (Vieira, 2015).

A Day in the Life of a Dementia Patient

Navigating through **mild dementia** can feel like you're a high-functioning pirate on a foggy sea. Your cognitive ship sails pretty well, but watch out for those little squalls that toss everything up in the air! Take getting dressed, for example. You might pop your T-shirt on inside out and strut around none the wiser. Or the morning coffee saga—no sugar bowl in sight could launch you into a frenzied treasure hunt through every cupboard, turning your kitchen into a scene right after a tornado.

You skip the coffee, clueless about the hurricane you just cooked up, and later, you swear up and down you had nothing to do with the mess. Insisting you're as innocent as a lamb while everyone else is sure you're the culprit? That's a surefire recipe for frustration and a bit of growling.

That's your daily groove: almost normal but always just a step away from mayhem. Old routines are your lifelines, but anything new? That's the monster under the bed. Ask about something from earlier, and it's a gamble whether your brain plays ball or plays hide-and-seek. By sunset, you're exhausted from these mental gymnastics, but sleep plays hard to get.

Your brain doesn't clock out; it keeps throwing puzzles at you like, "Where are my car keys? Must be stolen! Need them now!" leading to a wild goose chase at midnight, flipping through drawers like a mad hatter. The kicker? After all that hunting, you can't even remember what you were after. Oh, and a twist of fate—you haven't driven in five years. Welcome to the wacky world of mild dementia, where every day's an adventure, whether you remember it or not!

Moderate dementia takes everyday life and turns it into a series of pop quizzes with no warning. Think of it like being in your own mini-drama where simplicity is your co-star. Breakfast, lunch, and dinner aren't just meals; they're the main events of your day. Throw something new into the mix—like a rogue doctor's appointment—and it's like a storm hit your calm waters. Suddenly, your brain has to juggle more balls than a circus clown.

Take something as simple as a shower. To you, it's not just getting clean; it's like stepping into a different universe. The bathroom might as well be a space station with its cold, hard surfaces—a far cry from the cozy nooks you're used to. Disrobing feels like an episode of 'Naked and Afraid.' Then, the shower itself is like standing under a waterfall with an orchestra playing in the background, what with the hiss of water and the bombardment of soap, shampoo, and towels. Oh, and don't forget the unexpected cameo of someone 'helping' you, turning it into a full sensory overload show.

I once read about a guy in an assisted living home who described his first shower there as being cornered and pelted with rocks. That was his blockbuster interpretation of water hitting him. Another resident seemed to be taking part in a mystery movie, pacing hallways, dodging windows, and mumbling about avoiding 'Indian attacks.' It turns out her back pain from an old car crash felt like arrows hitting her, so naturally, in her screenplay, 'Indians' were the villains.

As words start to slip away, those around you become like amateur linguists, trying to piece together your sentences. When you don't understand others, it's like trying to crack a foreign language. Suspicion becomes your go-to emotion—because, honestly, if someone started giving you directions in Martian, wouldn't you be a bit wary?

Navigating moderate dementia, which often feels like the longest season of a very twisty TV series, is like wandering through a maze filled with land mines and dead ends, all populated by faces that seem increasingly less familiar and more like guest stars. But understanding the unique plot twists of this condition can help us all become better co-stars in this journey, armed with a bit more understanding and a lot of compassion.

Sliding into **severe dementia** is like sneaking into a movie theater; it's a subtle shift, barely noticeable until you're fully in the dark. The brain, heavily under renovation from the disease, no longer perks up at the sound of a favorite song. Instead, it prefers hitting the snooze button, turning life into an endless naptime.

Talking becomes like trying to catch fish with your bare hands—slippery and rare. You might cook up a whole speech in your mind, but when it comes to delivering it, you're lucky if a couple of words flop out. Caregivers become part-time detectives, piecing together these sparse clues. Vision gets all wonky, too, turning the world into a strange abstract painting.

I once read about a woman deep into her Alzheimer's journey who couldn't even recognize a puppy, let alone connect with it, despite her daughter's attempts to jog her memory with furry cuddles. Her passion for music? That ship had sailed, too. Her daughter would play her favorite musicals, but the response was as blank as a paused DVD.

In severe dementia, you're living in a perpetual 'now.' The past and future are like canceled TV shows—no longer airing. As you enter the final stages, it's mostly about catching Z's, turning waking life into a kind of hazy dream state where even making sense of a conversation is a rare event.

As this saga continues, eating transforms into an extreme sport, where even swallowing is a high-risk activity, possibly leading to aspiration pneumonia. Body functions downshift to slow-mo, and maintaining a stable body temperature becomes as tricky as predicting the weather.

In the end, your body waves the white flag, shutting down bit by bit, and sleep becomes your main hobby, leading you gently into eternal rest.

It's a tough ride, a real tear-jerker of a journey through the world of Alzheimer's-type dementia—and unfortunately, it's a script shared across the board with all types of people.

Can I Avoid Getting Dementia?

Sadly, there's no magic wand to banish dementia, and dodging its shadow is no easy feat. After the big reveal—getting diagnosed—you might get 8 to 10 years with your LOWD. But, as the saga unfolds, time becomes a fiendish character. As dementia advances, what remains is just a whisper of that once vibrant person. It's a tough pill to swallow, but any of us could find ourselves in this plot, especially if dementia runs in the family tree. Yet, all hope isn't lost.

Though it could quite possibly be too late for me, and I've come to terms with that, here's a secret for you, dear reader: You possess the power to tip the scales against dementia. Armor up with good self-care—physically, emotionally, and spiritually—to shield yourself from dementia's dark march. If you're currently in the caregiver's cape, resist the urge to neglect yourself amidst the chaos of stress or frustration. Shine the spotlight inward and nourish both body and soul.

Choose the path of health to boost your brain's defenses. Eat well, keep stress at bay, and nurture your mental health. **Aim for a life filled with balance, joy, and resilience**. Remember, while these steps don't make you invincible against dementia, they forge a stronger, happier, and more resilient you.

Steer clear of anything that might sabotage your well-being—be it mental, physical, or spiritual. Live a life true to yourself, one that enriches both your body and spirit and you'll definitely bolster your odds against dementia. And don't forget, the spiritual stuff matters too—it's all connected to your overall wellness. So, soak in this knowledge, knowing that each step you take today could be a giant leap for all your tomorrows.

Risk Factors Associated With Dementia

Imagine your health as the swashbuckling captain of a ship sailing through the choppy seas of life. You're the boss, the big cheese, and the decisions you make—especially about your lifestyle and well-being—are like setting the coordinates on your GPS. To steer clear of the stormy wrath of dementia, a tricky beast fueled by both your genes and the world around you, you've got to commit to a lifestyle that's as clean as a sailor's whistle on inspection day.

Sure, you can't dodge the aging process—it's like the ever-present ocean spray while you're at the helm. And yes, your family tree does throw some genetic coconuts in the way, but remember, they aren't the whole crew. Skimping on brain health or living like a pirate on shore leave can really tip your ship.

Don't underestimate the power of a good, brainy book or a health seminar. Keeping informed is like having the best navigational charts; it helps you avoid the Bermuda Triangle of bad habits and reduces your chances of hitting the dementia iceberg.

And what about the link between hearing loss and dementia, recently spotlighted by the brainy folks in lab coats? Losing your hearing isn't just about asking people to repeat themselves; it makes your brain work overtime, which can tire it out and even cause it to shrink. Plus, not hearing well might make you want to retreat from social gatherings, and that isolation is like throwing fuel on the dementia bonfire. Studies suggest that about 8% of dementia fog could be traced back to those missing sound waves (*Hearing Loss and the Dementia Connection*, 2023).

So, keep your ears sharp, your lifestyle sharper, and remember, while you can't control the wind, you can definitely adjust your sails.

Now, let's talk about those moody years in college. Turns out, being down in the dumps as a young adult might just boomerang back when you're 70-plus, messing with your cognitive sparkle and upping your odds for a dementia debut. And hey, it's a double whammy because depression can also crash the party as one of dementia's BFFs (Seladi-Schulman, 2022).

Next up in this festival of fun facts: loneliness. Not just the "forgot to invite me to the party" kind, but the hardcore, "I could win a gold medal in solitude" kind. This level of solo adventuring can spike your dementia risk by a staggering 50% and even fast-track you to the great beyond (*Loneliness and Social Isolation Linked to Serious Health Conditions*, n.d.).

And if you're a champion of the chair, beware. Lounging around like it's an Olympic sport can actually shrink part of your brain—the medial temporal lobe. Yes, the very place where your brain likes to stash its goodies. Thinning it out puts you on the VIP list for the dementia club starting midlife (Kiger, 2022).

So, what's all this doom and gloom good for? It's your cue to take the reins of your health and make some smart swaps. Understanding these risks isn't just a horror story—it's your toolkit for tweaking your destiny. By grabbing control of what you can, you're setting sail away from the rocky shores of dementia and towards a sunnier horizon. Let's lace up those sneakers, dial up the social calendar, and maybe even throw a little party for your brain. Why? Because getting through life isn't just about staying afloat—it's about cruising in style.

Ways to Delay Dementia

Seriously, though, the march of time inevitably brings changes to our bodies, with cells replicating and deteriorating as part of the aging process. However, there's good news: there are effective steps you can take to stave off dementia. Making lifestyle adjustments is crucial, not just optional, for those aiming to preserve their health and vitality as they age.

Remember, aging doesn't automatically mean you'll suffer from dementia or other cognitive decline diseases. But without guarantees, proactive action is essential. Here's how you can actively work towards delaying dementia (*Reduce Your Risk of Dementia*, n.d.):

- **Get Moving:** Lace up those sneakers and hit the pavement for at least 30 minutes of moderate sweat sessions on most days. Not only does it boost your brain juice, but it also keeps you from ballooning, which is great because being overweight is like rolling out the red carpet for dementia.
- **Eat Smart:** Stack your plate with fruits, veggies, whole grains, lean meats, and good fats. It's like giving your brain a spa treatment with every bite.
- **Social Butterfly Mode:** Keep your social calendar jam-packed. From garden clubs to ballroom dancing, staying connected not only spices up your life but also sharpens your wits, keeping those dementia gremlins at bay.
- **Health Check:** Wrestle down any party-crasher conditions like high blood pressure or diabetes. Mental health is part of the guest list, too—keep depression and stress checked at the door.
- **No Smokes or Soaks:** Ditch the smokes and cap the boozing. These bad habits crank up your dementia risk faster than you can say "cognitive decline."
- **Protect Your Head:** Whether you're biking or playing football, guard that noggin. A helmet can save your brain from taking hits that might invite dementia later.
- **Brain Gym:** Keep those neurons buff with continuous learning—books, online courses, you name it. Think of it as CrossFit for your cortex. (Cox, 2018)

Trudging through the maze to a dementia diagnosis isn't a walk in the park—it's more like a trek through a brainy jungle, complete with a variety of tests and evaluations. You'll meet a cast of characters along the way, from neurologists to geriatricians and even neuropsychologists, who are like the Indiana Joneses of brain exploration. They're the pros who'll help pin down that elusive diagnosis, and we'll dive deeper into their adventures in the next chapter.

Remember, arm yourself with knowledge—it's like having a superhero's toolkit. Getting a grip on these brain-busting strategies is a massive leap towards living a kick-butt life, no matter how many candles are on your birthday cake.

Chapter 2: Diagnosing Dementia: Unraveling the Clues

"Love keeps our memories alive, preserving their significance in every encounter, regardless of what we may have forgotten." –S.R. Hatton

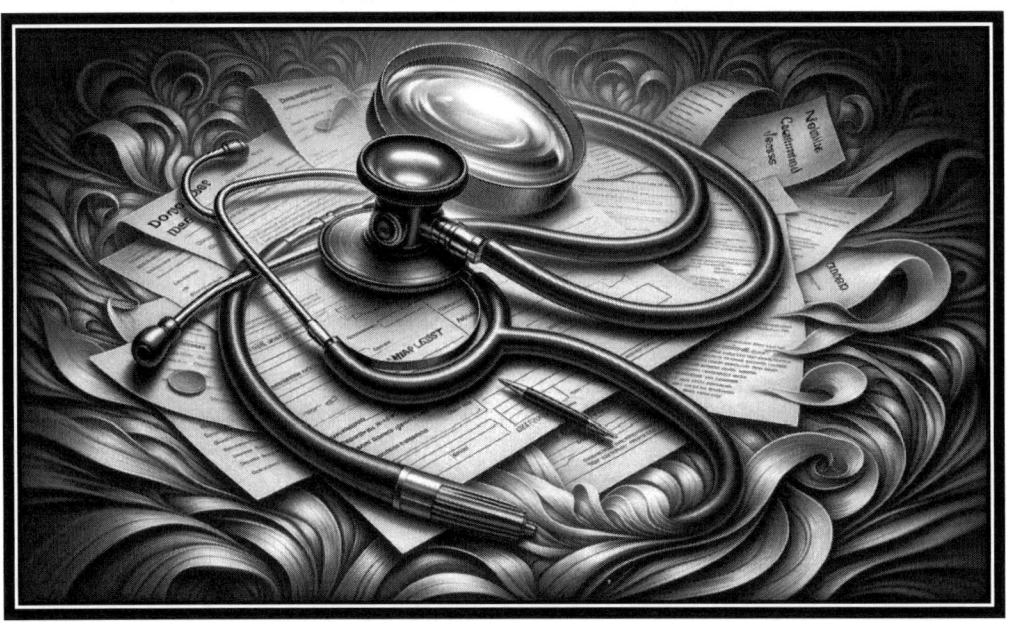

Opening Pandora's Box: Approaching the Subject of Dementia Diagnosis

Now, let's dive into the quirky world of Lesley and her mom. In the more silent moments of Lesley's life, her mom's odd habits started flashing like neon signs at a dodgy motel. The woman who once had her life color-coded and alphabetized began losing her keys to the mysterious voids of their home and leaving her purse behind like breadcrumbs in a fairy tale. She looped through stories like a broken record in the family room, and maybe even more eerie, she'd chat with ghosts—recalling dearly departed friends as though they were out grabbing a latte.

The real kicker was watching her mom, a whiz with any gadget from blenders to smartphones, suddenly eye the microwave with suspicion, like it was plotting her demise. And those ghostly heart-to-hearts? They were a stark, cold reminder of her slipping grip on the here and now.

Lesley, moonlighting as an aging parent coach while spearheading projects at a big pharma giant, found herself script-flipped into the caregiver role—a plot twist she hadn't seen coming. The thought of her mom duking it out with dementia? Scarier than any horror flick. With her professional life a demanding beast and her mom's antics setting off internal alarm bells, Lesley was torn between Excel sheets and existential dread.

Her workdays morphed into a juggling act, with her thoughts tiptoeing around mom's forgetfulness. Feeling the pinch, Lesley's gut screamed, "Doctor, stat!" So, off they went to a memory clinic, where after what seemed like enough tests to qualify her mom as a lab rat, the verdict was Alzheimer's.

As gut-wrenching as that label was, it gave Lesley something solid to stand on. Armed with this new, grim map, she could plot out the care her mom needed, making the unpredictable a tad more navigable (Lawrence, 2015).

And here we are, at the crossroads of diagnosis, gearing up for the trek through dementia. It's all about spotting the signs, keeping your cool, and remembering that knowing the beast is half the battle. Understanding dementia isn't just medical mumbo jumbo; it's your best weapon in keeping up the good fight, for you and your loved ones.

Hold up, I think this is a great spot to hit the pause button and dive into a treasure trove I stumbled upon—a YouTube goldmine for all things dementia. It's called Careblazer TV, where the brilliant Dr. Natali Edmonds drops knowledge bombs about the early warning signs and more. If you've been running around like a headless chicken looking for solid dementia advice, let me throw you a lifeline. Save those precious minutes for something else—like enjoying a good cuppa—and hop over to her channel, Dementia Careblazers. She's probably got answers to questions you haven't even thought of yet!

Careblazers TV on YouTube

For a quick sample, check out her six-minute scoop on early dementia warning signs right HERE. Trust me, it's time well spent.

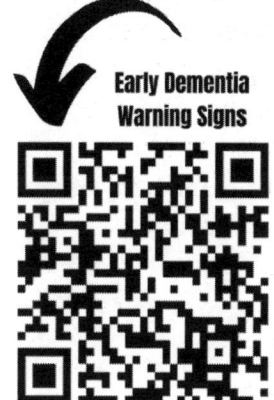

Early Dementia Warning Signs

Persuading Your Loved One to Get Tested

In the topsy-turvy world of dementia, your loved one might feel like they've accidentally stepped onto a rollercoaster—familiar things start looking alien, and regular routines get jazzed up into unexpected thrill rides. That's what Lesley found out with her mom, who was so fiercely independent she'd probably arm-wrestle you for the last cookie. Convincing her to get checked for dementia was like trying to argue with a cat; both frustrating and futile. Sometimes, you've got to call in the big guns, like a pro who can wave the diagnosis flag more convincingly.

Then there are times when your loved one sees the storm brewing and actually comes to you, spilling the beans about their struggles. But oh boy, there can be moments when they cling to denial like a stubborn barnacle on a ship, shrugging off the idea of a doctor's visit even as their memory starts throwing more errors than an old Windows PC.

In these wild waves, remember to keep the conversation flowing. Check in often. Chat about their day, lend a hand with chores, or just lend an ear. Show them you're their biggest fan, ready with a pom-pom or a pie, whatever helps. Ask them in a way that doesn't get their hackles up, like, "How do you feel like you're doing? Is everything as it has been, or are there things that aren't the same?" Their answer(s) could determine your next step.

Guide to Choosing a Doctor

If they're digging their heels in about seeing a doctor, maybe it's time to tag in someone they trust, like their GP, who can charm the socks off and gently nudge them towards testing. Just be cautious and don't try to rush the process because if the provider you choose misdiagnoses them, it will be much harder to persuade them to get tested again. (Check out this guide to choosing the right doctor to evaluate memory problems in your loved one from the Alzheimer's Association—it could be a game-changer for you.)

Another tactic would be to let your guard down and let the love show; sometimes, just knowing you care is enough to get them moving toward help. Your support could be the nudge they need to take that first big step to understand what's happening in their minds (*How to Get a Parent Tested for Alzheimer's and Dementia | Take Care*, n.d.).

The Path to Dementia Diagnosis

Now that I've got you brimming with resources that you'll need and want, let's get back to discussing the next step in this journey: getting an actual diagnosis. It starts with detailed discussions (with both your loved one and their doctors) and culminates in clarity, setting the stage for tailored treatment and coping strategies. Here is a glimpse into this multi-layered process (*Diagnosis*, 2018):

The Journey Begins with History: The process kicks off with questions about the patient's medical history, probing into past illnesses, and any significant events that might explain symptoms like stress or memory loss. These explorations form the foundation for distinguishing the type of dementia manifesting in the patient.

Physical and Mental Examination: The journey continues with a comprehensive physical exam and mental analysis. Expect inquiries about the current date, repetition of sentences, or even a challenge to count backward in a series of numbers. These simple yet critical tests help ascertain the patient's cognitive status.

Into the Labs: The exploration deepens with a series of lab tests, investigating the health of the thyroid gland, checking vitamin B12 levels, and conducting a blood count to screen for potential infections. Tests also check vital organs like the heart, kidneys, and liver to ensure they're functioning optimally.

Exploring Beyond the Surface: Further lab tests examine blood levels of electrolytes and glucose. Additional screenings include HIV tests, toxicology tests, and assessments of the patient's autoimmune system. Even the presence of heavy metals in the blood is investigated. A lumbar puncture may be performed to test for proteins in the spinal fluid, providing additional insights into the patient's health.

Imaging the Brain: The medical detective work extends to brain imaging tests, which help rule out other issues causing the symptoms, such as brain tumors. Tests include CT scans and MRIs—invaluable tools in the battle against dementia.

CT Scans and MRIs: These scans not only look for signs of strokes (linked to vascular dementia) but also help pinpoint the type of dementia, offering a more targeted approach to treatment.

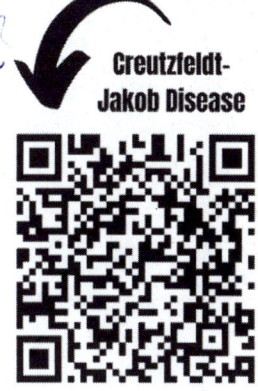
Creutzfeldt-Jakob Disease

Additional Testing: The quest for answers might entail further exploration of the brain's functionality. An electroencephalogram (EEG) can measure the brain's unusual activity, distinguishing dementia from other conditions. This test is also used to detect rare forms of dementia, such as Creutzfeldt-Jakob disease.

This diagnostic expedition is vital in defining the type of dementia a patient is facing, shaping the treatment path, and enabling everyone involved to better manage the ensuing journey with confidence and clarity.

Financial and Legal Planning—The Earlier, the Better

Wading through the complexities of financial and legal planning is especially tricky when dementia is in the picture. It's best to start early, while your loved one can still make clear decisions. Engaging a lawyer early on is crucial to draft the necessary documents, including granting you power of attorney. This legal step enables you to manage their finances and make decisions on their behalf if they become unable to do so themselves.

Approach these conversations with **sensitivity and persuasion, not force**. Your objective is to handle essential legal matters while your loved one is still lucid. As dementia progresses—sometimes accelerating quickly, without warning—it can become difficult for them to participate in these decisions, including crafting their will. Addressing these important issues while they are still legally 'of sound mind' ensures that their wishes are respected and legally protected (*How to Get a Parent Tested for Alzheimer's and Dementia | Take Care*, n.d.).

Finding your way through the intricate corridors of estate planning can feel like a maze with no exit. However, insightful, real-life advice can illuminate the path ahead. Let's dive into some hard-earned wisdom from another caregiver who has walked this path (and learned some hard lessons along the way), making it easier for you to follow. These are things that, at a minimum, your LOWD should have in place while they still have all their faculties intact:

1. **Assign Direct Beneficiaries:** Ensure your bank accounts have designated beneficiaries. When you pass, the beneficiary only needs your death certificate and their ID to access the accounts.
2. **Transfer on Death (TOD) Deed:** If you're a homeowner, consider filing a TOD deed with your county. This document allows you to transfer your home to a designee upon your death, saving your heirs a considerable amount in probate costs.
3. **Living Will:** This document states your wishes regarding healthcare decisions, especially when you're unable to communicate them personally.
4. **Durable Power of Attorney:** With this, you can assign someone to make legal decisions on your behalf if you're incapacitated.
5. **Power of Attorney for Healthcare:** This gives a designated person the authority to make healthcare decisions for you.
6. **Last Will and Testament:** This specifies the beneficiaries of your personal belongings.
7. **Funeral Planning Declaration:** Detail your preferred arrangements for your body and funeral services in this document.

8. **Consider Personal Care Agreements:** Caregiving often requires financial sacrifice. Formal personal care agreements can help compensate caregivers while addressing potential complications like Medicaid, tax issues, and family conflict. (An example agreement can be found HERE.)

In states like Michigan and Indiana, having these documents in place can help you avoid probate. Without them, you'll need to open an estate account at the bank, which requires a lawyer and invites potential claims on your property—a hassle you want to avoid!

Moreover, compile a list of all your financial accounts (including account numbers), credit cards, utilities, etc., and provide clear instructions on how to manage them. Ensure your heirs know where to find life insurance policies and have access to all crucial account logins and passwords (like Apple ID and bank account credentials).

Ensure you have titles for all properties, vehicles, campers, etc., in a safe and accessible location.

And perhaps most crucially, communicate your wishes to those close to you. Have open conversations with the people you've designated for various roles, as well as those you didn't. Explain the rationale behind your decisions to prevent misunderstandings or hurt feelings.

Unfortunately, our advisor shares that their father had intended to execute a TOD deed for their house but passed away before doing so, resulting in significant legal fees and a probate process. The hope is that sharing this experience can spark conversations and encourage everyone to take these crucial steps early on.

Remember, while these lessons are from personal experience and not legal advice, they should prompt a vital dialogue between you, your loved ones, and a professional who can help you navigate these crucial steps.

The intricate dance of caregiving is a delicate one, woven with legalities and emotions. For some additional fundamental steps that you should understand and master as a caregiver, follow this link to an article called *10 Must-dos When Serving as a Caregiver for Family.*

28 | Dealing with Dementia for Caregivers

Friends (due to copyright protection, I am unable to provide the details in my book). You might also want to check out the Commission on Law and Aging website for more comprehensive resources and information.

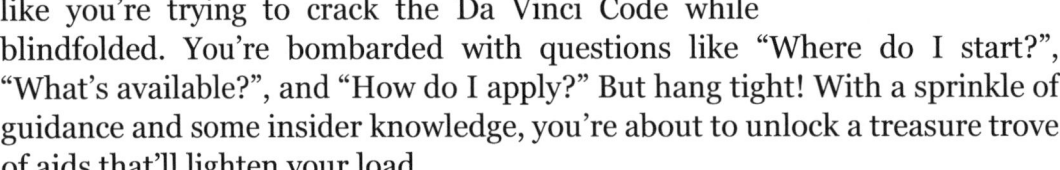

Bridging the Gap: Accessing Vital Support for Dementia Caregiving

Diving into the vast ocean of government and community resources for dementia care can often feel like you're trying to crack the Da Vinci Code while blindfolded. You're bombarded with questions like "Where do I start?", "What's available?", and "How do I apply?" But hang tight! With a sprinkle of guidance and some insider knowledge, you're about to unlock a treasure trove of aids that'll lighten your load.

Let's first decipher the array of resources. From financial relief and medical care to support groups and sanity-saving respite services, there's a lot on the table. For instance, Medicaid can ease the financial burden of healthcare, while local community centers might offer support groups for camaraderie and shared advice.

> *As of 2024, 46 states and Washington, D.C., offer some level of assistance for individuals in assisted living or other forms of non-nursing home, residential care through their Medicaid programs (Cobb, 2024). (PayingforSeniorCare.com)*

The secret to unlocking these resources lies in knowing the right places to look. Your first port of call? Try your local Area Agency on Aging (aka the Eldercare locator), which is like Central Command for services such as meal delivery, transportation, and caregiver support programs. The Alzheimer's Association also offers comprehensive guides on accessing these services.

Tackling the application process can feel daunting—kind of like trying to assemble a spaceship with a screwdriver. Equip yourself with all the necessary documents—medical records, financial statements, proof of residence—to streamline this process. If you hit a snag, don't hesitate to call in reinforcements from social workers or senior organization representatives.

But there's more to it than just signing up. For instance, don't just use respite care to catch a break; maximize it to rejuvenate and return to caregiving with renewed energy. Active participation in support groups or workshops can also bolster your practical skills and emotional resilience.

And let's not overlook the power of advocacy. Stepping into this role can seem intimidating, but it's a potent way to shape the broader discourse on dementia care needs and policies. By joining advocacy groups, participating in awareness campaigns, or sharing your experiences with policymakers, your efforts can help mold a more dementia-friendly society.

Congrats on making it this far! As a reward for your stellar endurance, I've whipped up a free downloadable guide packed with all these resources (and a few extra surprises). Think of it as your ultimate connection cheat sheet. Grab it, use it, and thank me later. Access it here: *Lifelines for Dementia Caregivers*.

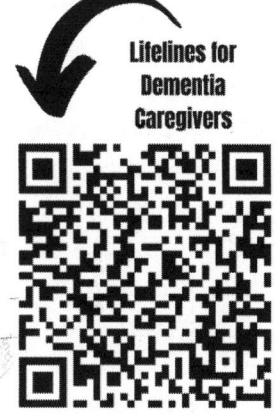

And please don't be afraid to dive into the treasure chest of resources I've stacked up for you because, let's face it: Knowing is only half the battle—the real magic happens when you roll up your sleeves and actually use them! By tapping into these goodies, you boost your caregiving superpowers and join a league of extraordinary supporters. This isn't just about upping your caregiving game; it's about plugging into a network that has your back, ensuring you're never flying solo on this wild ride. Get in there, get connected, and show 'em how it's done!

The Emotional Impact of a Dementia Diagnosis

Managing the emotional whirlwind after your loved one's dementia diagnosis is intense. It feels like you're trapped in the most dramatic reality TV show ever. But don't fall into a pit of self-pity, especially while your loved one can still join in on family jokes and recall sweet memories. Getting swallowed by sadness now might lead to regrets later when the disease throws more curveballs like hallucinations and weird delusions.

Instead of wallowing, why not open up a space where your loved one can share what's on their mind? After all, they're facing a pretty big life change, and it's only right to let them express their feelings, fears, and bucket list dreams. This isn't just your journey—your loved one's voice is super important, too.

By keeping things gentle, you can help them share their worries and hopes, building a zone of trust and love. As things get twistier with their disease, your loved one will lean on you more and more for care and understanding. They'll need you to be their superhero—someone who can bring a bit of calm to their confusing new world.

So, gear up with loads of empathy and patience. Your mission is to be there for hugs and reassurance when things get scary for them. And while you're saving the day, remember you're not flying solo. There are plenty of other 'sidekicks' out there—people just like you, figuring out how to care for their loved ones. Don't forget to take care of yourself, too. After all, even superheroes need a break!

Banner Alzheimer's Institute

Now, let's cut to Dr. Pierre Tariot, the veteran showrunner at the Banner Alzheimer's Institute, with over 35 seasons—err, years—of experience. He's seen many cast members (i.e., dementia sufferers) frozen by fear, worried they'll lose their lines or forget their cues, as their cognitive abilities start to fade. It's a common myth that an Alzheimer's diagnosis is the series finale, causing too many to cancel their subscriptions to treatment after just a few episodes.

Here's the shocker: more than half of those with dementia exit the show early, never even knowing they were part of the cast—they miss out on the critical plot developments that early detection and treatment can offer. Yes, you read that right. Over 50% of people with dementia die **without ever knowing they have it**—meaning they never understood how to deal with it! This lack of awareness costs them more than just plot holes; it robs them of a chance to manage symptoms effectively and plan for future seasons (Tariot, 2019).

So don't just passively watch this series unfold for your loved one. Use the available resources, connect with the supporting characters, and maybe even write a few episodes yourself. After all, being proactive can turn what seems like a horror show into something a bit more manageable—maybe even a dramedy (which is sort of how I view this book. Hey, if I can't beat it, I'll join it and try to help others like me in the process!).

I'd also like to pass on some expert strategies to help you navigate these tricky emotional waters:

Let It All Out: Think of your emotions as steam in a pressure cooker—it's better to vent than to explode. Crying isn't just acceptable; it's practically recommended!

Ride the Emotional Rollercoaster: Some days; you're the hero and other days; you're the sidekick who fell in the mud. Roll with the punches. A crummy day today could be a setup for a comeback tomorrow. Cherish the good days, and on the bad ones, remember what got you through.

Embrace Your Inner Drama: There's no "correct" way to feel. Feeling a smidge resentful or wishing you were anywhere but here? Guess what? You're not alone, and it's totally normal.

Talk It Out: Whether it's unloading onto a friend or confiding in a pro like a Dementia Adviser or an Admiral Nurse, getting those messy feelings out can help you untangle them.

Write It Down: If talking isn't your style, try writing. Scribble in a diary, pen a letter to your future superhero self, or draft unsent letters to vent. It's like giving your brain a good declutter, making room for more positive thoughts (Alex, 2023).

I also want to add one more: **Appreciate empathy.** Recognize that your feelings stem from a place of great compassion. These traits show your ability to empathize with others' experiences. View your role as an opportunity to serve your loved one and others in similar circumstances. Find a purpose in your new situation, transforming it into a blessing for others.

Up next, we'll explore some of the more puzzling complexities of dementia by hearing some heartfelt stories from other caregivers who share essential tips for managing challenging situations like hallucinations and sundowning (with as much compassion as possible)

Chapter 3: Real-World Advice for Major Caregiving Hurdles

"Choose truth over denial, for even in the darkest of moments, eternal happiness resides—fueled by the everlasting power of love." —S.R. Hatton

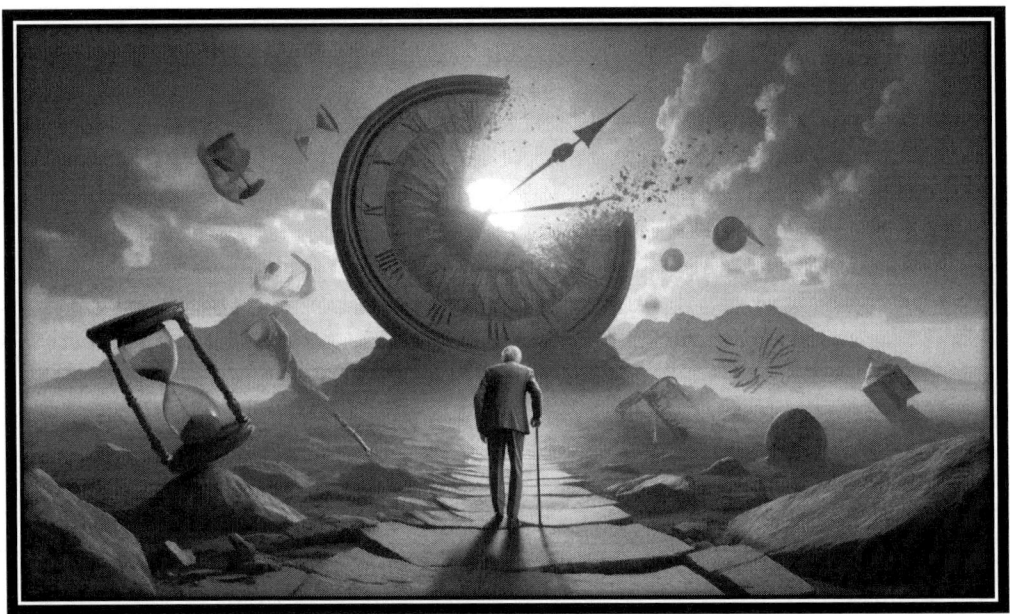

Heartbreak and Hallucinations

Every visit Meg Wilkes made to her husband Keith's nursing home room was a harrowing heartache, a poignant reminder of a love story challenged by the relentless march of dementia with Lewy Body. For years, Meg had been grappling with the heart-wrenching decision to leave Keith in a nursing home, confined to a single room but surrounded by the 24-hour care his worsening condition demanded.

In her seventies, Meg wanted nothing more than to care for Keith at home, but his needs had grown too profound. He required assistance with everything—from bathing and dressing to eating and navigating his wheelchair—not to mention the exhausting tasks of managing the surreal and often distressing hallucinations that had become Keith's reality.

These days, Meg's visits to Keith were always laced with profound sorrow. On one visit, Keith announced, with hopeful tears, that he had fully recovered, inspired by a television program on stem cell research. Another time, he solemnly told her that one of them had passed away, but he wasn't sure who. His hallucinations ranged from believing Meg was conspiring with the care staff to witnessing dead infants lined up on his bed. These delusions left Meg floundering, unable to piece together any logic, yet she held on and listened, trying to provide comfort.

Meg's heart ached as she remembered their life together before the nursing home, when delusions had already started invading their home. Once, while Meg was away for the weekend, Keith had been found in a church, tearfully telling a friend that Meg had died. He had imagined their son was battling AIDS, a delusion that persisted for a full month. Then there was the prolonged saga of the imaginary letter. For months, Keith searched every nook and cranny of their home, convinced that Meg was hiding this crucial piece of correspondence. He even wanted to dismantle the house, believing the elusive letter was hidden behind the skirting boards.

Meg watched, helpless and weary, as dementia took her husband to places she could never reach. She clung to their memories and tried to find solace in their past, even as dementia's cruel grip continued to pull Keith further away.

Yet, while pushing through this ongoing storm of confusion, one poignant moment stood out for Meg—a moment every caregiver holds dear when it happens. During a rare lucid interlude, Keith, aware of his delusions, expressed his gratitude to Meg, his sole source of coherence. His words brought Meg immense relief, affirming her decision not to indulge in his delusions but to provide a stable, grounded presence.

Meg cherished that lucid instant. It was the only time Keith seemed truly himself, a fleeting moment of recognition, love, and awareness. The cruel irony of Lewy body dementia is that most of the time, loved ones don't recognize their caregivers as they once did. The disease twists perceptions, turning love and familiarity into estrangement. It doesn't matter if you're a spouse, child, or parent; dementia sneaks up when least expected, following its inevitable course.

The affliction tormented both of them, but Meg gradually found acceptance. She had already mourned her husband long before his physical departure. It was as though Keith had been imprisoned within his own body, a living shell holding the essence of someone already lost (Wilkes, 2018).

To Pretend or Not to Pretend

I'm guessing you've already realized that the wild and unpredictable landscape of dementia care isn't for the faint-hearted, nor does it come with a one-size-fits-all rulebook. Carol Bradley Bursack knows this all too well, having cared for her father and several other family members. She's braved the maze of contradictory advice and found a surprising ally—pretending (also referred to these days as "validation theory").

Carol's journey with her father sheds light on this controversial aspect of dementia care. Torn between two doctors, one who scolded her for indulging her father's delusions and another who praised her for it, Carol faced a conundrum. Then came the breakthrough: her father's unwavering belief that the University of Minnesota had forgotten to send him his medical degree. Instead of fighting this delusion, Carol crafted a counterfeit degree, complete with his name and some scribbled signatures. Hanging this faux diploma on her father's nursing home wall brought a light to his eyes—his long-awaited degree had finally arrived.

With experience spanning the care of six family members and even a neighbor battling dementia, Carol's advice is golden. Should you always pretend with dementia sufferers? That's a personal call, a balancing act each caregiver has to master. But Carol emphasizes one crucial point: arguing against their delusions can do more harm than good. Instead, listen compassionately, offer assurances when they're scared, and let them know they're safe. In the topsy-turvy journey of dementia care, kindness, understanding, and empathy are your true north.

So, whether you're faking diplomas or just lending a compassionate ear, remember: there's no right or wrong way, just the way that brings peace and comfort to those you love. After all, if you can't beat dementia, you might as well get creative with it (Cpmi, 2014).

Shedding Some Light on Sundowning

Now, let's discuss a phenomenon that's as common as bad karaoke—sundowning. You may have already noticed that as the sun sets, your LOWD transforms. The calm person you once knew suddenly becomes agitated, and your familiar world takes on a bizarre twist. Welcome to sundowning, a wild ride every dementia caregiver must learn to tame.

The timing and intensity of sundowning can vary, but if you're not prepared, your evenings can quickly become a wicked roller coaster ride. Picture yourself frantically trying to settle your LOWD while they insist on rearranging the entire house at 10 PM. Sounds fun, right?

Learning about sundowning is crucial, and there's no better way than by listening to the tales of others in the same boat. Take this gem from an anonymous caregiver: "My mom starts pacing like she's training for a marathon, swearing and fiddling with the lights. Getting her to bed is like wrestling an octopus." Or the one who said, "At 9 PM, my mom suddenly turns into Sherlock Holmes, searching for 'clues' and making tea. Is this sundowning?"

Though challenging, understanding sundowning is vital for caregivers. Recognizing it and learning its key manifestations can help turn your nightly chaos into a more manageable experience. As the sun starts to set, watch your LOWD for these specific behaviors:

Restlessness: Picture your loved one morphing into a hyperactive squirrel, endlessly pacing or fidgeting with anything they can get their hands on—like rearranging the living room for the tenth time that day.

Agitation: Imagine someone as jumpy as a cat on a hot tin roof, constantly uneasy and on edge, ready to react to the slightest disturbance.

Rage: Think of a peaceful bunny suddenly turning into the Hulk, experiencing extreme anger or hostility over the smallest things, like a misplaced TV remote.

Irritability: Your once patient loved one now gets frustrated quicker than you can say "Netflix buffer," snapping at minor inconveniences like a slow internet connection.

Confusion: Their usual level of daily confusion gets cranked up to eleven, leaving them puzzled about their surroundings, like wondering why the kitchen sink isn't in the living room.

Suspicion: They develop unfounded beliefs of mistrust, convinced that the mailman is plotting to steal their prized collection of rubber bands.

Delusional behavior: Holding onto clearly untrue beliefs, like insisting they're the long-lost heir to a forgotten kingdom that doesn't actually exist.

Demanding things: Imagine a broken record of insistent and repetitive requests, asking for items or actions over and over—like demanding the "good ol' days" be brought back immediately.

Upset moods: Prolonged periods of sadness or disinterest, like Eeyore on a particularly gloomy day, showing little enthusiasm for anything.

Anxiousness: Persistent worry, nervousness, or fear, like they're constantly waiting for a test they didn't study for, even if the only test is figuring out what's for dinner.

Recognizing these symptoms and learning how to respond to them is like mastering a tricky dance. Sundowning may be heartbreaking to witness, but understanding it can empower you to provide the most compassionate and effective care for your loved one.

Supporting Your Loved One Through Sunset

Navigating the challenges of dementia, particularly during the disorienting hours of sundown, can feel like you're herding cats in a thunderstorm. But armed with these tips, you can significantly reduce the discomfort and anxiety often experienced by your LOWD at twilight:

- **Familiarity is comforting**: Keep their surroundings as consistent as possible. It helps them feel secure.
- **Provide comfortable sleeping arrangements**: A different bed or bedroom might make them feel safer. Keep night lights on in key areas to avoid any midnight mishaps.
- **Embrace their rhythm**: Accept their skewed body clock. Help them figure out if it's breakfast time or bedtime.
- **Avoid stress**: Sidestep stressful situations and conversations, like dodging potholes on a bumpy road.
- **Promote tranquility**: Keep your home as peaceful as a meditation retreat, especially when they're around.
- **Maintain calm**: Avoid heated conversations near them. They don't need to be in the front row of your drama.
- **Provide space**: Understand their struggle to distinguish dreams from reality. Be their anchor in the storm.
- **Monitor their energy**: Note their sleep patterns. If they're up at night, think nocturnal owl, not party animal.
- **Involve their doctor**: Discuss their sleep issues with a healthcare pro for tailored advice.
- **Understand their patterns**: Bc aware that dementia can cause them to feel more energetic at night than during the day.
- **Prioritize self-care**: Stay rested. Your exhaustion can unintentionally trigger their suspicion.
- **Recognize triggers**: A confusing day can lead to a chaotic night. Keep their day as predictable as a clock.

To make evenings smoother, try these real-world strategies:

- **Plan for the day**: If possible, schedule activities, appointments, and personal care for the morning or early afternoon.
- **Structure routines**: Stick to consistent wake, meal, and bedtimes.

Real-World Advice for Major Caregiving Hurdles | 37

- **Embrace the sunlight**: Get them outside during the day for a dose of sunshine.
- **Keep a journal**: Track their behaviors to spot patterns and triggers.
- **Reduce evening stimulation**: Minimize TV, chores, and loud noises in the evening.
- **Balance meals**: Big lunch, light dinner. Think of it as dietary feng shui.
- **Brighten the home**: Ensure good lighting in the evening to reduce confusion with strange shadows.
- **Soothe with activities**: Engage them in relaxing activities, like listening to calming music.
- **Promote relaxation**: Offer gentle massages or calm conversations before bed.
- **Keep them company**: Stay with them during restless moments, offering soothing words.
- **Offer reassurance**: Remind them you're there, like a comforting lighthouse in the fog.
- **Coordinate medication**: Discuss the timing of medications with their doctor, especially around sundowning.
- **Limit daytime naps**: Especially if they struggle to sleep at night.
- **Avoid certain substances**: Keep them away from alcohol, nicotine, and caffeine.
- **Seek medical guidance**: Consult their doctor for potential solutions to the toughest situations.
- **Approach gently**: Stay calm and loving if they're upset, agitated, or angry.
- **Be attentive**: Ask what they need and do your best to provide it.
- **Avoid confrontation**: Arguments will only escalate anxiety and anger.
- **Reinforce support**: Constantly reassure them of your support and love.
- **Allow movement**: Let them pace if they need to, but keep a watchful eye.
- **Avoid physical restraint**: Unless absolutely necessary, and even then, tread carefully.

Patience and empathy are your best allies. By simply understanding what's happening to them, you can be the light that guides them through the darkness of sundowning (Morrow, 2023).

Sundowning Advice from Caregivers

Sandra K. would hear her mother's voice every night around 8 pm, like clockwork. Restlessness would seize her mother, a woman who spent most days nestled in the quiet corners of idleness. She would ask Sandra to pray with her, their hands intertwined, voices raising a soft hymn to the heavens. At the prayer's end, her mother would smile, a glint in her eyes, and say, "I hope you're right!" The two would share a laugh, a brief bubble of warmth before the chill of night set in. Sandra would tuck her mother into bed, a ritual she now yearns to relive, if only for one more sundowner.

Teresa F. has weathered the stormy seas of sundowning, and if there's one beacon she can offer, it's calmness. She firmly believes in loving them through it, in giving solace through soft words and patient reassurances. She urges fellow caregivers to grant their loved ones the space they need during sundowning, even as the heartbreak claws at their hearts. Be a constant presence, a tranquil balm, and reassure them that even as the sun sets, they are not alone.

Becki S. dances to a different tune during sundowning, a tune infused with fun and warmth. With her mother, she spins games from the threads of imagination, bringing laughter into their twilight hours. The two have embarked on countless adventures, journeys within the confines of their home during sundowning. Now, fun is an inseparable part of their routine. Becki's advice is this—step into their world, immerse in their perceptions, and allow them the freedom to be themselves during sundowning.

Shawn W. kept a small basket of socks and hand towels in his mother's room that 'needed to be sorted.' When she'd wake in the night feeling restless and disoriented, this simple (and not overwhelming) task that 'needed to be done' gave her something familiar to do until she became sleepy again. It also provided her with a sense of purpose and kept her from wandering out of her room at all hours of the night.

Tereasa C. infuses her mother's sundowning hours with soothing rhythms and calming visuals. She swears by the healing power of music, its notes wafting through the room like an unseen comforter. She also enjoys using calming videos to engage her mother and diffuses essential oils to create an ambiance of absolute tranquility.

As we transition into the next chapter, we'll uncover even more strategies for caring for those living with dementia. Every challenge in caregiving is a lesson waiting to be learned, and understanding these common pitfalls can turn your journey into a more fulfilling and rewarding experience. So, let's dive in and discover how to make this journey a little smoother and a lot more meaningful.

Chapter 4: A Caregiver's Guide to the Galaxy

"Embrace the unraveling of life's threads, for it is through this delicate dance of chaos that your soul begins to weave a beautiful pattern of purpose and growth." –S.R. Hatton

---

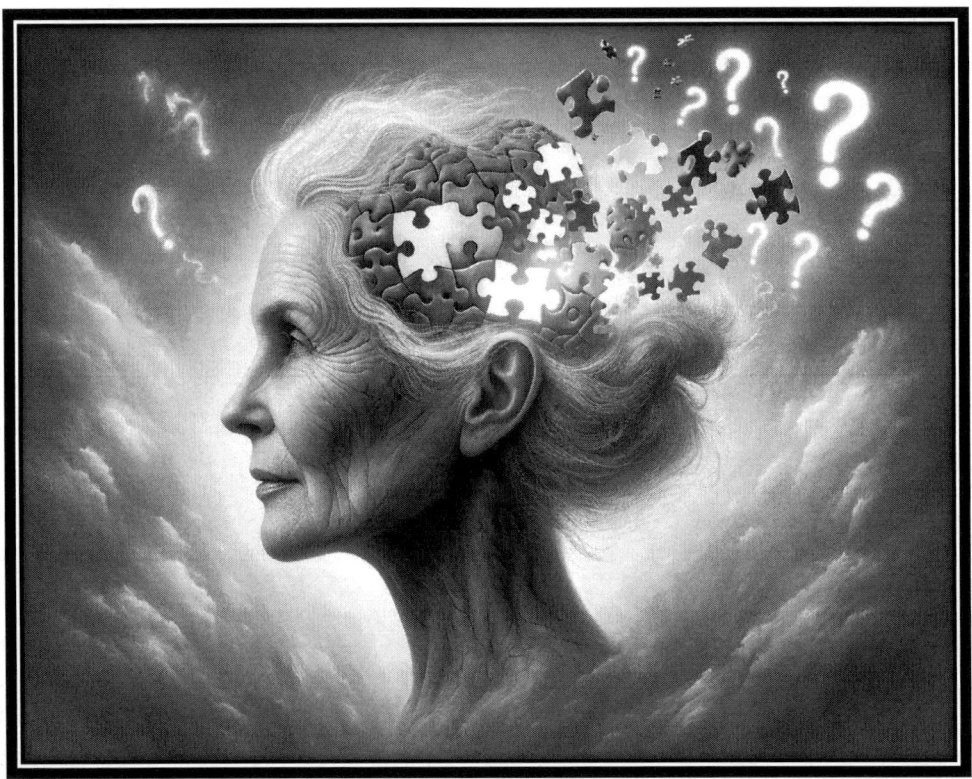

Sweet Acceptance: Embracing Gratitude and Releasing Bitterness

Despite the tides of dementia chipping away at his mother's cognition, Joseph refused to believe she was lost to him. The echoes of "Your mom is gone" bounced off him, leaving no impact. His mother's core—her essence of love, compassion, and care—remained steadfast, a beacon of her presence. Once a dedicated caregiver herself, a woman who poured love and kindness into her family, neighbors, churchgoers, and anyone who craved a tender touch, she was not one to be erased by an ailment. Her words might have betrayed her, but her actions spoke volumes.

The nursing home staff, now her caregivers, reported instances of her helping others at the home. It was then that Joseph's belief was reaffirmed; his mother was not gone. She was there, radiating love in her unique, silent way. Her moments of tranquillity were woven into the fabric of her caregiving nature.

Admittedly, when her memory clouded their names, bitterness snuck in. The proclamation, "She's not there, she doesn't love us," echoed through their hearts. However, Joseph soon realized it was their bruised egos reacting, yearning for acknowledgment from a mind trapped in a fog. But she was present; she communicated love wordlessly. For instance, her restless fidgeting stilled when Joseph's dad sat beside her, lulling her into a peaceful sleep in her chair. Joseph reflects, "Those who said she was gone were wrong. What remained was her most genuine self." (Creamer, 2018)

Caring for a loved one with dementia is a round-the-clock commitment that can often stretch your limits. When the weight becomes unbearable, seeking professional help isn't a sign of failure, but rather a commitment to ensuring safety and adequate care for your loved one. The decision to hire a caregiver or resort to a nursing home might seem daunting, but remember, it's an act of love, not defeat.

Families like Joseph's have walked down this path, choosing to place their loved ones in nursing homes as the disease progressed. On the other hand, many opt for home care, a choice gaining popularity. Out of the 5.8 million people diagnosed with dementia in the United States, most are cared for at home (*Dementia Care: Keeping Loved Ones Safe and Happy at Home*, 2024).

If you find yourself facing this daunting task, know that you're not alone. This book, the expanse of online resources, and the supportive network of professional carers in your community or online can offer invaluable guidance. Counsel from qualified medical professionals and experienced caregivers can transform your approach to challenging situations, turning seemingly insurmountable obstacles into surmountable hurdles.

There's Always More to Learn

You've been a trooper, journeying with me through this complex maze of understanding dementia and the nuances of caregiving. As we go deeper into this expedition, it's crucial to remember that there's always more to learn, and with experience, wisdom will grow. Home caregiving, as you're probably realizing by now, is no stroll through the park. It's a puzzle filled with complexity and an intricate dance of ensuring safety and comfort for your loved one.

In the upcoming chapter, we'll delve deeper into the physical modifications your home may need, because any little thing could stir the waters of peace and amplify their vulnerability. It's your mission, your calling, to furnish the highest standard of care that your loved one deserves, turning each challenge into a victory. And yes, the path may get rocky, as dementia often brings escalating demands. That's why planning ahead, like a caregiver executive, is the key to sustainable success and mitigating the risk of burnout or chronic stress.

Don't just see yourself as a family member, but envision yourself as the CEO of a caregiving partnership who carries out tasks diligently, faithfully, and with honor and dignity. There are some crucial tenets to keep in mind as you wear this hat:

> **Provide comfort and reassurance**: This is the lifeblood of your relationship with your loved one. Offer them a soothing presence, a tender touch, a compassionate heart—even when recognition fades from their eyes. It's not their fault; don't take it personally.
>
> **Striking the balance**: Navigating the space between helping them and respecting their dignity is essential. Let them wander within the safe confines of your home or enjoy the tranquility of the garden. Give them room to breathe, and simultaneously lighten your load.

Dancing Through Dialogue: Tips for Effective Communication

When conversing with someone experiencing dementia, it's like stepping into a slow dance—so here are some essential rhythm steps to learn that will keep you both moving smoothly:

1. **Speak in Bitesize Beats:** Like you're explaining the rules of checkers to a five-year-old, use short sentences and clear words. For example, instead of a soliloquy on why we wear hats, try, "Hats keep your head warm!"
2. **Eye Contact Tango:** Lock eyes like you've spotted a rare bird. This helps them focus and feel valued. Imagine you're trying to spot that bird without scaring it away.
3. **Pause for Applause:** Give them the stage. Rushing them to finish a sentence might make them feel like they're being pushed off it. Think of it as waiting for the microwave—patience brings the reward.
4. **Group Chat Jamboree:** Encourage them to mix it up at social gatherings, like a quiet mixer, not a rave.

5. **Solo Speeches:** Let them be the star of their own show when it comes to their care discussions. Think of them as the COO making the big operational decisions in your caregiving partnership.
6. **Respect the Mic:** Avoid patronizing. No one likes a comedian who bombs by laughing at their own jokes instead of the audience's reactions.
7. **Acknowledgment Encore:** If they go off-script, show you're still engaged. It's like nodding along to a jazz solo that has wandered off the melody.
8. **Choice Choreography:** Offer them simple this-or-that choices. Like choosing between vanilla or chocolate ice cream, not the 31 flavors at Baskin-Robbins.
9. **Creative Communication:** If words fail, try rephrasing. It's like changing the salsa music to a slow waltz to match their steps.
10. **Patience Polka:** Stay calm and patient; it sets the tempo and makes the communication flow more smoothly. Imagine you're teaching someone to dance for the first time.
11. **Cheerful Chatter:** Keep your tone light and friendly, like a Disney character greeting park guests.
12. **Respectful Space:** Chat at a comfy distance, maybe sit if they are sitting, making it feel like a relaxed coffee chat rather than a tense job interview.
13. **Hand-Holding Harmony:** Sometimes, a gentle touch can be reassuring, like holding hands during a scary movie, but always watch for cues if they prefer more space.
14. **Engaged Eye-Contact:** Encourage them to look at you, reinforcing that you are both present in the conversation—like you're both focusing on the same interesting painting at a gallery.
15. **Don't Cut the Line:** Avoid interruptions, even if you anticipate their thoughts. It's not a race to finish each other's sentences.
16. **Focused Attention Foxtrot:** Dedicate your full attention by turning off the distractions—like muting the TV during the final game-winning play so you don't miss a beat.
17. **Feedback Waltz:** Repeat what they say for clarity, like an echo in a valley, ensuring you both heard the same thing.

These steps aren't just dance moves; they're ways to ensure each interaction is as clear and joyful as possible, keeping the rhythm of your communication smooth and respectful (*Communicating With Someone With Dementia*, 2023).

With all that said, wouldn't it be awesome to have a list of tips and reminders that you can print out and stick somewhere handy? Like the back of the bathroom door where you hide and have a good cry on those overly stressful caregiving days? Well, here it is!

Survival Cheat Sheet for Dementia Caregivers

Alert: This ain't your doctor's prescription, just a sprinkle of my own experiences and hard-learned lessons from actual caregivers. (In other words, this is not to be taken as medical advice, just real-world advice from people who do this every day).

1) Channel your inner tortoise! Speak slowly and steadily and lock those peepers when you talk. (Maintain eye contact)

2) Master the art of Zen focus. Just one thing at a time, it's all about keeping the confusion at bay.

3) Choices, choices, choices… Keep it simple, cap their choices at two.

4) Simplicity is the ultimate sophistication. Stick to yes/no questions, one-sentence instructions, and maintain that eye-to-eye connection.

5) Double is your new favorite number. Whether it's bath time, mealtime, or just a general task, give yourself twice as long to get things done.

6) Deal with tantrums as though they're a toddler in the 'terrible twos' stage: Stay cool, whatever they do, just "let it go." Use distraction and switch their focus. KISS (Keep It Simple, Silly) it! Be clear and calm and use simple language without trying to reason with them or argue—it's like trying to negotiate with a teddy bear!

7) Become a memory magician. If outings are still in the cards, recreate their favorite haunts for an experience full of nostalgia.

8) Be a sensory explorer! Revisit activities they used to love that tantalize all five senses, from their favorite sights to the most delicious tastes.

9) Turn on the sound of music! Blast their favorite tunes, better yet, the ones that you both used to rock out (or sing) to.

10) Dehydration is a known enemy to dementia sufferers! Water is like the oil to the engine of our bodies, and if your loved one isn't getting enough of it, they could experience amplified symptoms. Dehydration can lead to

especially when health and safety concerns grow. Maybe their solo shopping trips need a rethink, or you might just need to spend more time with them. The goal is to keep as much of their main routines as possible, even as things evolve.

Here's a great example: Jed Levine, the CEO of Caringkind, a non-profit supporting seniors and dementia caregivers in New York City, shares a story about a family transitioning their mother to a new care environment. The mother was initially agitated, struggling to adapt. Then, her daughter had a stroke of genius: every Sunday, they handed her the New York Times—a longtime habit. And voila! She found peace flipping through the paper, even if she didn't fully understand the articles (Botek, n.d.).

The takeaway from this tale is that keeping familiar habits can be a soothing balm for their frazzled minds. If your loved one enjoys playing the piano, schedule time for it and encourage it! Offer their favorite teatime snacks, reminiscent of happier times. Let them watch their old favorite TV shows in the afternoon. By replicating the rhythm of their past life, you can help boost their mood and rekindle their joy.

Navigating the dementia maze isn't just about managing symptoms; it's about cherishing the individual and celebrating their unique story. So, as you plan each day, remember—your mission is to bring moments of comfort and happiness to their world, one routine at a time.

Creating a Personalized Checklist of Enjoyable Activities

As you draft the daily game plan for your loved one, picking the right activities is crucial. Mix it up with both active and passive engagements they can enjoy solo, with you, or with other seniors—it's therapeutic gold. The secret sauce? Each activity should light them up with joy and give them a sense of purpose—something they actually look forward to.

Whether it's dusting off old hobbies or trying out new interests, the goal is a day full of meaning and fulfillment. Not sure about a new activity? No worries—give it a whirl and see if it's a hit before making it a staple. To help you nail this activity plan, here are some nuggets of wisdom:

Make it Personal: Think of their favorite hobbies as a GPS for activity planning. Love fishing? Dust off the old rod. Passion for knitting? Yarn it up!

Cultivate Joy: Monitor their reactions like a hawk. Are they smiling or scowling? Their emotions are now your guide to success.

Harness Skills and Abilities: Draw from their past. Got a former chef? Let them stir a pot or two. A retired gardener? Hand them some seeds and let the magic grow.

Prioritize Safety: Transform their environment into a safe haven. Do they love gardening? Ensure the backyard is escape-proof and slap on some sensors to avoid any Houdini acts.

Celebrate the Journey, Not the Destination: It's about enjoying the ride. If they're having a blast, who cares about the outcome? Focus on fun, not perfection.

Encourage Self-Expression: Unleash their inner artist! Painting, piano, knitting, or just jamming to some tunes—let them express themselves. Introduce simple group games for some social sparkle.

The magic of meaningful activities is like a secret superpower. As you plan their day, think beyond just keeping them occupied. Aim for moments that spark joy, unleash creativity, and fill their world with fulfillment. And don't worry about trying to fill up every minute with an activity. Ample time for breaks and resting should also be included depending on your LOWD's condition—as well as an enormous amount of flexibility on your part. Their mood and stamina will fluctuate often, so be ready to change it up at a moment's notice if need be (*Daily Care Plan*, n.d.).

Activity Ideas to Include in Your Daily/Weekly Planner

1. **Encourage Cognitive Stimulation:** Engage their minds with activities like crossword puzzles, reading, or simple chores around the home. These activities aren't just time-fillers, they're valuable tools for brain stimulation. (One suggestion: Unlock precious moments of connection and nostalgia by immersing your loved one in my companion book, *Tales from Memory Lane: Large Print Short Stories for Seniors with Dementia & Fans of Easy Reads*. With each turn of the page, embark on a journey through memorable events and extraordinary individuals, igniting the spark of engagement and reviving cherished memories.)

2. **Craft a Food Diary:** Create a dining schedule featuring their favorite meals while keeping nutrition in check. Picture them enjoying grandma's famous chicken soup—good for the soul and the body!

3. **Make Cooking a Collaborative Affair:** Bring them into the kitchen! Mixing cookie dough or preparing a salad can be a delightful, brain-stimulating bonding experience.

4. **Foster Participation in Household Tasks:** Let them help with making tea or setting the table. It's a small but mighty way to make them feel accomplished, especially in the early stages of the disease.
5. **Prioritize Personal Hygiene:** Schedule routine self-care activities like baths, haircuts, and nail care. It's not just about cleanliness; it's a boost for their dignity and self-esteem. Think spa day vibes at home!
6. **Celebrate Their Hobbies:** Whether it's knitting, painting, or gardening, weave these hobbies into their weekly routine. Watching them light up as they plant flowers or knit a scarf is pure gold.
7. **Don't Skip a Beat with Medication:** Create a foolproof medication schedule. Picture an elaborate system with alarms, pillboxes, and maybe even a choreographed reminder dance—anything to keep them on track!
8. **Cultivate Social Connections:** Plan regular visits with friends, family, and social groups. Picture the joy of a Sunday brunch or a family BBQ—social ties are a lifeline for emotional comfort and cognitive health.
9. **Plan Excursions and Holidays:** Schedule outings to their favorite places from the past. A trip to the old family cabin or a beach day can bring comfort and joy, offering a refreshing change of scenery.
10. **Promote Physical Activity:** Incorporate daily exercise like park walks or gentle garden yoga. Think of it as their personal vitality-boosting routine, enhancing mood and health.

Remember, these activities are more than just tasks—they're essential steps to ensure your loved one's well-being, fulfillment, and dignity. And they're not just beneficial for them; they're also unique opportunities for you to connect, engage, and create meaningful memories together.

Exploring Unconventional Therapies for Your Loved One

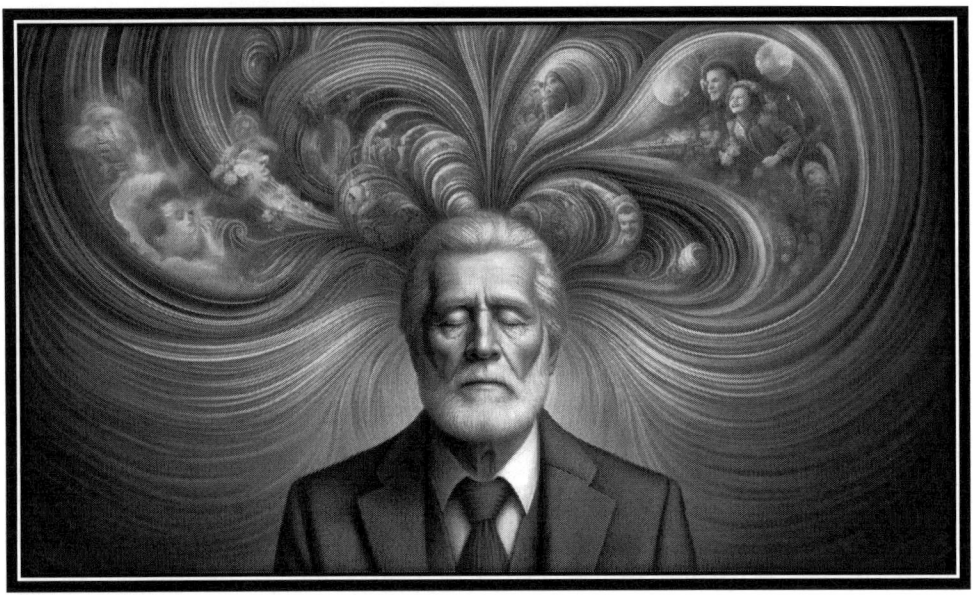

Reminiscence and Life Story Work

Alright, if you're ready to dive deeper than just strolling down memory lane, let's embark on an epic quest with your LOWD—crafting a Life Story file! This project isn't just about capturing memories; it's like assembling a highlight reel of their greatest hits. Rekindling these moments not only bolsters their sense of identity but also keeps their dignity shining bright. With roots in reminiscence therapy, this technique is a powerhouse for lifting spirits and boosting overall well-being.

Following the sage advice of Dementia UK, creating a Life Story file isn't just a nostalgic trip—it's a strategic move. This file becomes a treasure trove of invaluable info, helping others understand and care for your loved one better than ever. Curious how to start this heartfelt journey? Well, keep reading because I'm very excited to tell you all about it!

Understanding the Life Story

Think of the Life Story as your LOWD's personal highlight reel or a mini-biography, packed with all the juicy (and important) details. It's an intimate collection that jogs their memory, fosters a deeper understanding of your loved one, and **becomes a priceless tool for caregivers and health pros**. Plus, creating one is a delightful activity to tackle together or through professional reminiscence work. Let's take a look at the awesome benefits:

- It's like a reflective road trip through their life.

- It reinforces their sense of personal identity—no ID required.
- It brings comfort through familiar memories and moments, like a cozy blanket of nostalgia.
- It strengthens bonds with family, friends, and caregivers, like a super-glue for relationships.
- It equips social care workers with essential information about their identity, preferences, and needs—no more guessing games.

Building the Life Story File

You can let your creativity soar while creating this repository of memories with your loved one.

- **Create a Photo Book:** Assemble a vibrant book filled with photos, using contrasting colors and simple graphics. Remember to avoid patterns, as these can be confusing for dementia patients. (According to a *Good Housekeeping* article in April of 2024, the best overall photo book maker is Shutterfly, and the best-themed photo book maker is Mixbook.)
- **Design Collages:** Piece together a visual narrative using their favorite and most memorable photographs. (These are some of the best-rated programs on the web to create your own collage masterpieces: Pic Collage, one of the best for new users because it guides its users with instructions and on-screen tutorials; Instasize, highly rated because it offers a generous collection of filters, borders, layouts, etc. without having to purchase the premium version; and Canva is also a great option with lots of free templates to choose from. Actually, Canva is what I used to help create all of the QR code images throughout this book.
- **Embrace Technology:** Video recordings are a wonderful medium to capture dynamic memories. Consider creating a documentary-style video, allowing them to voice their thoughts, wishes, and heartfelt messages to family and friends. (One suggestion: check out my other

companion book, *The Memory Keeper: A Guided Journal for Recording & Preserving the Life Story of Your Loved One with Dementia,* for this exact purpose. A collection of nearly 100 thought-provoking questions, it includes fun and unconventional prompts to guide you in creating a video documentary capturing the essence of your loved one's life. Or you may choose to forego the video documentary and record all of your loved one's answers in the journal itself. Not only will you capture valuable information crucial for their care, but you'll also create a timeless keepsake for future generations to cherish. I do hope you'll give it a whirl…I put my heart and soul into making sure it includes all the important questions, as well as some that no one has ever thought to ask before—which makes it lots of fun!)

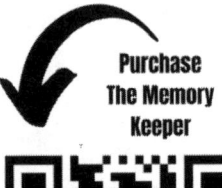

- **Assemble a Memory Box:** Collect personal items that hold special meaning for them. A memory box for a person with dementia should contain items that evoke powerful emotions. Consider incorporating objects that engage all five senses—sight (photographs of friends and family or a video of themselves talking about their life), taste (a favorite candy bar or other treat), touch (objects from a favorite hobby like a golfball, yarn, or a favorite shirt or pajamas), hearing (a CD or other recording of their favorite music), and smell (favorite body lotion, perfume/cologne, or bar of soap), to craft an effective and sensory-rich keepsake box.

    Pinterest has some great ideas for making your own memory box (or purchase one from an online shop), but another great idea I ran across is to create an Online Memory Box that can be shared with anyone and everyone and will last forever. Check them out at Klokbox.com.

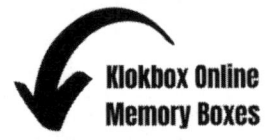

- **Compile a Personal Profile:** Capture comprehensive details about their life journey, including their career, birth details, parents, medical conditions, and other relevant information. (Note: *The Memory Keeper* also has a full chapter dedicated to compiling all of this important information for your loved one.)

Strategies for Success

Here are some pro tips to make the project smooth and enjoyable:

Team Up: Work closely with your loved one. Think of it as a fun buddy project where their stories and your curiosity make the perfect duo.

Stay Excited: Be enthusiastic, proactive, and adaptable. Channel your inner cheerleader and be ready to pivot if things get tricky.

Bite-Sized Chunks: Break down the process into manageable topics. It's like assembling a puzzle one piece at a time rather than dumping the whole box on the table.

Easy Does It: Avoid overwhelming them; pace the process to their comfort. Nobody likes a drill sergeant barking orders, so keep it chill and relaxed.

Break Time!: Take frequent breaks and create an enjoyable atmosphere. Play some background music, have snacks handy—make it a cozy memory-making session.

Memory Jogging: Gently prompt them to retrieve memories about people, places, photographs, and experiences. A little nudge goes a long way—like, "Remember that time at the beach?"

Feel Their Feels: Empathize with their experience and be sensitive to their needs. Be the emotional sponge, soaking up their stories with genuine care and understanding.

Essential Inclusions

Your loved one's Life Story file is like a greatest hits album, packed with all the essentials. Here's the lowdown on what you need to include, with a bit of flair:

Personal Details and Significant Relationships: Think of this as the "About the Author" section. Include names, birthdays, the inside scoop on family drama, best friends, and those frenemies they'd love to forget but can't. This helps everyone know who's who in their life's soap opera.

Childhood Memories and Work History: Capture those nostalgic moments when life was all about candy and treehouses, and then transition to their superhero-like career tales. Whether they were a mad scientist or a world-class knitter, every job has a story.

Major Life Events and Significant Places: This is the highlight reel. From that epic prom night to the unforgettable vacation in Paris, and even the time they tried bungee jumping (or at least thought about it), these moments are golden.

Fashion Preferences and Favorite Clothing Items: Document their style evolution. From bell bottoms and tie-dye tees to that one hideous Christmas sweater they adore, it's all about capturing their unique fashion journey.

Dietary Requirements and Favorite Foods and Drinks: Include everything from the "no peanuts" warning to their love affair with chocolate cake and the secret family recipe for meatloaf. Don't forget their favorite drink, whether it's a fancy latte or just plain old tap water.

Medical History Excluding Dementia: List all those medical escapades—surgeries, allergies, that weird rash they got in '97—everything. This helps caregivers navigate any medical minefields without stepping on a landmine.

Daily Routines and Favorite Entertainment Choices: Think of this as the script of their day. From morning coffee rituals to that 3 PM nap; don't forget their favorite TV shows, movies, or the book they read for the thousandth time. It's all about the rhythm of their day.

Hobbies and Regular Activities: Whether they're into birdwatching, Sudoku, or attempting to crochet an entire zoo, jot down all the activities that bring them joy. This helps keep their days filled with purpose and fun.

Other Daily Preferences and Important Lifestyle Details: Capture all the quirks and habits. Do they need three pillows to sleep? Prefer their toast slightly burnt? Love a good foot rub after a long day? These little details make all the difference in their comfort and happiness (Dementia UK, 2024).

Remember, this isn't just any 'ol exercise; it's a celebration of your LOWD's life journey. Think of it as their own personal blockbuster biopic, complete with laughter, tears, and the occasional plot twist. It's a living document that brings joy, enhances understanding, and, most importantly, restores a sense of dignity to your loved one's life. So, dive into this incredible journey of reminiscing and enjoy the shared experiences and stories it brings to light. It's like creating a family movie night, but with a lot more heart!

Guided by the Mind: A Revolutionary Dementia Therapy

So, picture this: The power of hypnosis, often seen as a parlor trick or stage show gimmick, is now stepping into the spotlight as a promising tool in dementia care. This practice, already a staple in the British therapeutic toolkit, is being cleverly used to help dementia patients and their caregivers. Let's dive into the mesmerizing world of hypnosis and see how it can work its magic on dementia.

Guided Hypnosis: Imagine it as a chill-out session led by a maestro, where you're gently guided into relaxation with soothing instructions and calming music. The internet is bursting with guided hypnosis tracks for just about anything you can think of.

Hypnotherapy: This is where the pros come in. Run by licensed doctors and psychologists, it's like the Swiss Army knife of therapy, tackling anxiety, depression, eating disorders, and other mental health gremlins.

Self-Hypnosis: Think of it as a DIY stress-buster. This technique lets you tap into the power of your mind to ease pain and manage stress, all by yourself (Cherry, 2022).

Armed with a basic understanding, let's talk about the groundbreaking world of hypnotherapy for dementia—a lesser-known trail that's already getting rave reviews in the UK and is catching on in the U.S. for dementia patients and their caregivers. First things first; remember that this is not medical advice, but I believe it could be a game-changer for many of us who are at the end of our ropes after seeing some of the curveballs this disease throws at us.

Back in 2007, Simon Duff and Daniel Nightingale, both esteemed researchers in dementia, revealed the transformative potential of hypnotherapy (Duff & Nightingale, 2007). Their comprehensive study showed that dementia patients who underwent hypnotherapy displayed better concentration, memory, and social skills. They were more relaxed and actively engaged in activities. Even the caregivers who got hypnotherapy showed a boost in their caregiving prowess.

Feedback from the study was overwhelmingly positive. Patients seemed calmer, happier, and enjoyed better sleep—even those in the advanced stages of dementia. Here are some key benefits:

1. **Enhanced Relaxation and Overall Demeanor**: Picture your loved one going from frazzled to Zen master. Hypnotherapy can turn the dial down on their stress levels, making them feel more at ease.
2. **Improved Concentration**: Think of it as a mental tune-up. Hypnotherapy helps sharpen their focus, so they're not wandering off mentally or physically as much.
3. **Greater Levels of Independence**: Imagine them reclaiming a bit more of their autonomy. Hypnotherapy can boost their confidence to handle daily tasks on their own.

4. **A Surge in Motivation**: It's like giving their drive a shot of adrenaline. Suddenly, they're more interested in participating in activities they used to enjoy.
5. **Better Short-Term Memory**: Picture them actually remembering where they left their glasses. Hypnotherapy helps improve short-term recall, making daily life smoother.
6. **Increased Socialization Leading to Less Isolation**: Visualize them chatting away happily at a social event. Hypnotherapy encourages social interaction, reducing feelings of loneliness.
7. **Improved Recollection of Significant Life Incidents**: Imagine them sharing a cherished memory from their past. Hypnotherapy helps them tap into their personal history, bringing joy and connection to their lives (Medical Hypnosis with Roger Moore, 2023).

Now, picture this: Me, wading through a sea of dementia articles, when suddenly, this nugget of gold glistens in the chaos. This next gem of wisdom is so priceless, it's like finding a cheat code for dementia care. Trust me, this little-known resource is about to revolutionize your approach to caregiving for your LOWD. It's time to blast this discovery to everyone on the dementia roller-coaster—the warriors battling it and the superheroes caring for them.

Enter Mr. Roger Moore, a hypnotherapy expert in California. Having completed his training with Dementia Therapy Specialists, he's now weaving the magic of neuroplasticity hypnosis into his practice. Roger's venture is turning out to be a blockbuster hit, with clients and their dedicated caregivers sharing stories of remarkable progress and improvement. (Moore et al., 2007).

The ultimate goal of his work is to flip the script and transform a life overshadowed by dementia into one blooming with REMENTIA. Yes, you heard that right, **rementia**—a jaw-dropping phenomenon where lost cognitive abilities make a comeback—basically putting dementia into remission! Dementia doesn't have to be the end; it can be the start of a different, but still meaningful journey.

Hypnosis offers the promise of a better quality of life for those living with dementia and their caregivers. Imagine a magic carpet ride where the magic is real, and the destination is wellness.

And here's the best part! **Free** (as of this printing, at least) **hypnosis consultations** for those affected by dementia are just a call or click away. You can book these at Palm Desert Hypnosis with Roger Moore or enjoy the comfort of your own home by connecting with him online through his Hypnosis Health Info Virtual Office. Reach out with any questions to 760-219-8079 or Roger@HypnosisHealthInfo.com. This could be your first step toward embracing the remarkable marvel of 'rementia.'

Even if this sounds like a wild idea, or you just aren't sure whether your LOWD is up for such an unconventional experience, I encourage you to search the internet for more information about the connection between dementia and hypnosis. There's new info popping up every month. From what I've discovered, hypnotherapy is indeed shaking up the dementia care world, bringing rays of hope, optimism, and tranquility to patients and caregivers alike.

(Another side note: For those of you wanting to try more mainstream styles of therapy for your loved one, such as cognitive behavioral therapy (CBT), I've included some links to information on that in my *Lifelines for Dementia Caregivers* handout.)

It's Not Just for Your LOWD

It's crucial to understand that hypnotherapy isn't just a beacon of hope for those grappling with dementia—it also shines its comforting light on carers, partners, and family members. Often burdened by fatigue, stress, and frustration as you tirelessly care for your loved one with dementia, don't be surprised if hypnotherapy helps you and other family members struggling to come to terms with their new reality find solace and rejuvenation after just one or two sessions.

Think of dementia as a cryptic journey into another 'dimension.' Despite the original meanings of 'dimension' and 'dementia' not intertwining, the idea weaves a poignant narrative. It paints a picture of our dear ones traversing unseen worlds, momentarily touching our reality in those fleeting, lucid moments. Like my grandma Bonnie, who, over time, seemingly inhabited a world distant from mine—most of the time, during her last years, she believed that she and my grandpa were 'on vacation in Missouri.' Far from the nursing home in Florida, where her physical presence was, it warmed my heart knowing that wherever she was, her mindset was that she and her dear husband were having a great time 'on vacation.' However, your LOWD may not have such pleasant throw-back memories, and coming to terms with this fresh reality demands patience and strength.

Remember, as caregivers, you're walking this path, too. The distress of watching your loved ones change, the lurking fear of our own susceptibility—we're strapped into an emotional roller coaster that doesn't seem to have a stop button. But guess what? There is a bit of hope within our reach—hypnotherapy.

There are so many ways that hypnosis and hypnotherapy can help you as the caregiver—the list is quite extensive. In addition to dementia and Alzheimer's, the other areas of medical hypnosis include:

Aging
Autoimmune Disease
Cancer
Chronic Pain
Dentistry
Depression, Low Self-esteem
Diabetes
End-of-life
Fibromyalgia
Headaches & Migraines
Hypertension
Irritable Bowel Syndrome
Parkinson's Disease
Sleep Disorders
Smoking Cessation
Stress Management, Anxiety, Phobias
Weight Loss

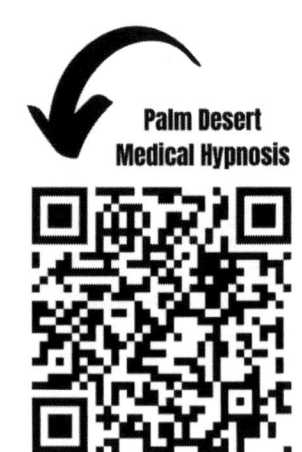

Palm Desert Medical Hypnosis

Hypnotherapy can help you tackle these issues head-on, and then some. It's like having a mental Swiss Army knife for handling the emotional heavy lifting of caregiving—in conjunction with any professional medical treatment you may need, of course. Here's how it can reshape your world (Palm Desert Hypnosis, 2020):

Healing Past Trauma: For some, the person under their care might have been part of a traumatic experience from their past. Hypnotherapy allows you to journey back, confront these emotions in a secure space, and reshape old, negative self-perceptions into new, empowering ones.

Managing Anxiety and Fear: Emotional awareness opens doors to understanding our reactions, enabling us to self-soothe when required. In other words, we learn how to keep our cool when things get really tough.

Letting Go of Anger and Sadness: Hypnotherapy provides a safe haven to address the uneasy yet natural emotions we encounter when caring for a relative with dementia. It offers a therapeutic avenue to vent anger, maybe towards the cared-for individual, absentee relatives, or even higher powers. Moreover, it gives you the freedom to express your sadness, shedding liberating tears that can help alleviate the emotional pain.

Focus on Self-Love and Self-Care: Hypnotherapy emphasizes rewriting old narratives and cultivating affirmations that celebrate self-love and positivity. Each session incorporates healing aspects, allowing clients to nurture their inner child and replenish fragmented parts of themselves, such as trust, courage, and self-esteem.

Hypnotherapy is indeed a formidable ally in aiding millions living with or affected by dementia in various forms. By unearthing the unconscious, it allows individuals to identify their struggles swiftly and address them on a profoundly deeper level than conventional talk therapy.

This isn't just therapy; it's a heart-to-heart journey into the deepest corners of your being, guiding you toward peace, understanding, and, most importantly, self-love. Embrace it, explore it, and let it illuminate your path as a caregiver.

Now, as you turn the page on this chapter of your caregiving journey, brace yourself. We're about to redesign your living space into a fortress of tranquility and familiarity for your loved one. Get ready to transform your home into the ultimate dementia-friendly retreat. The journey of a thousand tweaks starts with a single step—or page-turn.

Make a Difference with Your Review

Unlock the Power of Generosity

"Acts of giving are like potato chips: it's tough to stop at just one, and they're surprisingly good for the soul." —Anonymous

Imagine this: every time you laugh at a joke, somewhere, a fairy gets its wings. Alright, maybe not, but here's something equally magical—people who give without expecting anything in return often find themselves happier, healthier, and inexplicably better at trivia games. Why? Because karma is real (and possibly subscribes to your newsletter).

So, let's have a little fun while doing some good. I have a quirky request for you...

Would you help someone you've never met, even if the only reward was an invisible pat on the back from the universe?

Think of this mysterious person as your doppelgänger from another caregiving dimension. They're a bit like you were back when dinosaurs roamed the Earth—okay, not that long ago, but back when you first started caregiving. **They're hungry for guidance**, eager to make a difference, but as lost as a sock in a laundry cycle.

My mission is to arm every dementia caregiver with superpowers (well, the bookish kind, since I can't actually grant you the ability to fly or become invisible). Everything I do, every word I write, is fueled by this mission to reach, help, and empower.

That's where you, dear reader, swing heroically into the picture. It turns out that most humans do indeed judge a book by its cover (and what others say about it). So, **here's my whimsical plea on behalf of a caregiver you've never met**: *Please leave a review for this book.*

Your review doesn't cost a dime and takes less than a minute to write, but it **could be the secret ingredient** in another caregiver's victory potion. Your words have the power to:

- **Transform Confusion into Clarity**: Shed light on how this book is helping you decipher the maze of dementia caregiving.
- **Empower with Practical Magic**: Point out those chapters that were more helpful than finding a 20-dollar bill in an old coat pocket.
- **Foster a Band of Allies**: Every review helps build a fellowship of caregivers, turning solitary quests into a mighty, united front.

It's super easy: Just zap yourself over to the Amazon review page by scanning the QR code below with the camera of your smartphone and unleash your inner storyteller.

Thank you for adding your magic to the spellbinding world of dementia caregiving. Remember, your review could be the pep talk someone needs on a particularly dragon-filled day. Please consider sprinkling a little more joy and wisdom on the world, one review at a time.

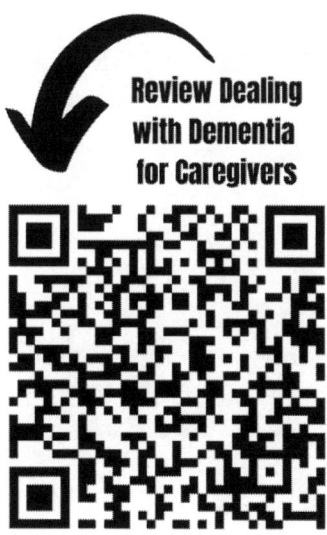

Chapter 5: There's No Place Like Home

"Love is not just a noun to be felt, but a verb to be lived; it provides us the courage to hold steady, even when the familiar fades into the unknown." –S.R. Hatton

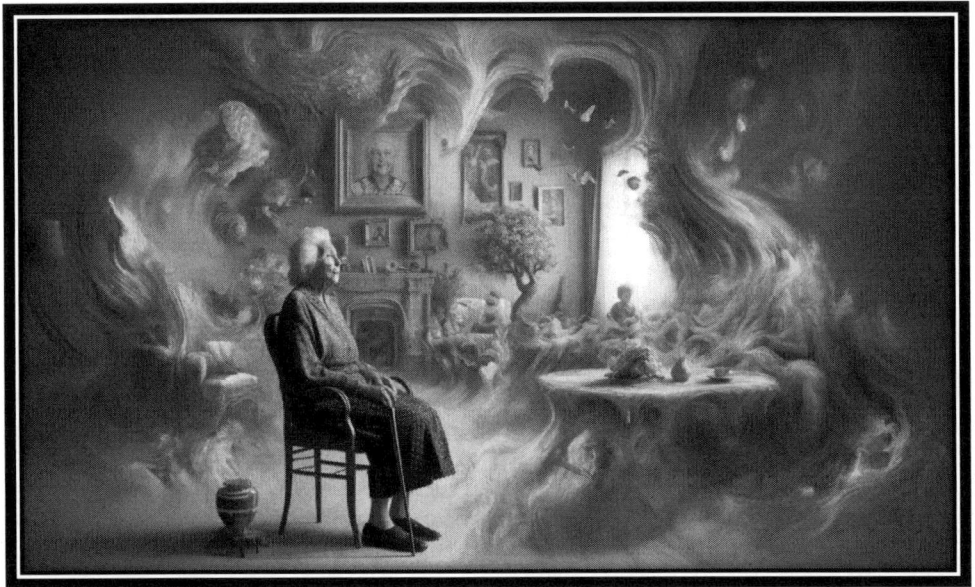

The Vulnerability of Dementia Sufferers in Their Own Backyard

Let's talk about a frustrating game of hide and seek that no one signed up for—Getting Lost Behavior (GLB). It's like trying to navigate through your hometown where all the street signs are suddenly written in alien hieroglyphs. GLB is a real challenge in the world of Alzheimer's Disease (AD), snagging about 40% of patients in its confusing clutches. And as the disease progresses to what we might call the boss level—severe AD—the odds jump to a staggering 70%. The stakes? Higher than just losing at hide and seek. We're talking institutionalization, the danger zone of falls, and even the ultimate game over: death. Despite GLB being a frequent flyer in the AD travel itinerary, scientists are still scratching their heads about why this happens. So, as much as we know about its impact, the real brain buster—the 'why' behind GLB—remains AD's little secret (Yatawara et al., 2017).

In the whimsical world of dementia, everyday settings can feel like a baffling game show where the paths change unexpectedly. Joe learned this firsthand during leisurely strolls with his mom, acting as her personal guide through the neighborhood—kind of like a low-budget travel show host, guiding her gently along the way and introducing her to familiar landmarks to keep her world from spinning out of control. Then, one fateful day, a phone call took his attention from her for only minutes, leaving his mother to navigate the suddenly alien surroundings. A harmless alley transformed into a vortex of confusion for her, making her mutter in a mix of fright and befuddlement, "This doesn't look familiar. Where am I? This isn't the way back home."

A stranger, briefly mistaken for Joe, became an unwitting lifeline in her sea of disorientation. The relief she felt when Joe reappeared could rival the joy of finding your car in a crowded mall parking lot during Black Friday. Once home, ordinary things like stairs suddenly morphed into Everest. With Joe's help, she tackled this 'mountainous' challenge, her breathing as heavy as if she'd actually scaled a peak. The next day, brewing a simple cup of tea turned into an 'Iron Chef' challenge, with ingredients and instructions slipping through her mind faster than a slick contestant evading capture.

Navigating the twilight zone of dementia involves turning everyday living into a supportive stage set, where every prop and cue is placed to guide and reassure. It's about making their home a sanctuary where familiar tasks are no longer daunting. This isn't just a care strategy; it's about creating a backdrop for daily victories in a world where reality often flickers in and out of focus.

Building a Dementia-Friendly Home: Colors, Patterns, and Consistency

As carers for loved ones with dementia, we often have to navigate the tricky path of blending our worlds. Their reality, sometimes fraught with confusion and clouded by delusions, hallucinations, and optical illusions, can seem distant and detached from ours. A simple yet effective way to bridge this divide is by creating a dementia-friendly environment at home, which can significantly ease their daily experience.

Bright, contrasting colors can be a beacon of clarity in the otherwise foggy maze of their perceptions. Such hues aid in distinguishing different objects and locations, making the house more navigable. Take your front door, for instance. Painting it a vibrant red can serve as a memorable landmark, helping your loved one recognize their home when stepping in or out.

Yet, while bright contrasts are friends, intricate patterns and stripes can turn into foes. These designs might induce disorientation or even cause anxiety. So, it's best to keep decor simple—plain and contrasting colors against the walls, ceilings, and floors. Ensuring furniture stands out is also crucial, which might mean replacing patterned or striped upholstery with solid colors.

Moreover, we must resist the urge to frequently rearrange furniture or redecorate rooms. The layout should remain familiar and consistent, fostering a sense of security and stability for your LOWD. Avoid having side tables or other furniture obstructing walkways, ensuring safe and unhindered movement.

Here, familiarity trumps aesthetics. If pictures, mirrors, and intricate designs confuse or frighten them, consider removing these elements. The same goes for bed linens; they should be brightly colored without complex patterns, providing a comforting contrast against the walls.

Practical Home Tips

Embrace armchair comfort: Choose chairs with armrests and avoid backless designs. Not only are these cozier, but they also aid in getting up and provide better stability. Ensure these seats are of an appropriate height to further ease the process.

Clear the pathways: Keep side tables and similar furniture pieces out of main walking areas or room centers. A clear, unobstructed path is the safest way to navigate the home.

Minimize visual confusion: Consider removing pictures and mirrors, especially from common areas and rooms frequently used by your LOWD. Reducing potential sources of confusion can offer them a more peaceful environment.

Consistency is key: Keep the home layout identical day in and day out. Consistent surroundings can be comforting and provide an incredibly valuable sense of familiarity.

Resist the urge to redecorate: During your loved one's stay, avoid the temptation to give your home a makeover. Let the place remain familiar and consistent, ensuring everything stays in its designated spot.

Highlight utilities: Light switches and appliances should contrast sharply with the walls. Clear visibility can help them locate and use these essentials with relative ease.

Say no to patterns: Avoid furniture featuring stripes or intricate patterns. Simple, solid-colored pieces work best in a dementia-friendly home.

Embrace contrast in bed linens: Choose bright, solid-colored bed linens that contrast with the wall. The simpler, the better.

Guide with green: Houseplants can serve as subtle indicators, guiding them toward the garden or other outdoor spaces.

Doorway to clarity: Painting doors in bright colors can help differentiate between rooms, making it easier for them to navigate their home.

Remember, the goal is to create a sanctuary that offers comfort, familiarity, and navigational ease for your loved one. Their home should be a space that caters to their unique needs and minimizes potential confusion, providing them with a sense of independence and tranquility.

The Art of Dementia-Friendly Flooring

Keeping your loved one with dementia safe is like baby-proofing your home for a remarkably tall toddler with an affinity for exploration. You need a clear path because anything, even that stylish rug you love, could become a booby trap. Throughout this book, I've been the bearer of not-so-great news: folks with dementia are, basically, magnetically drawn to incidents.

Those rugs you adore for their aesthetic value? They're actually floor banana peels waiting to happen. You might want to declare a "rug prohibition" to keep things smooth and uneventful underfoot.

Dementia has a way of remixing visual perceptions. A normal staircase could look like a ladder to another dimension. An interesting pattern could morph into a disorientating maze. Even shiny floors can seem like a treacherous ice rink; water on the floor could transform into a terrifying pit.

For peace of mind, keep your décor simple. Opt for plain, non-glossy floor coverings that don't turn into optical illusions. Here's how to spin your home into a dementia-friendly space:

Color coding: Wherever possible, the floor color should contrast with the walls and stairs. This helps to delineate spaces clearly.
Rug-free zone: Remove all floor rugs and mats to ensure a smooth, tripping-free surface.
Carpeting simplicity: If you opt for carpeting, choose plain colors that contrast with the walls for easy differentiation.
Tidiness is safety: Keep all wiring and cables out of sight. If they can't be hidden, ensure they're securely fastened and don't pose a tripping hazard.
Staircase visibility: Highlight the edges of stairs with bright paint, tape, or stair edging. This makes each step clearly visible, reducing the risk of missteps.

I realize that some of these tips are just not practical to implement—we can't always remodel our home to fix the flooring issue, for example. But, every tweak and adjustment you **can** make is a step toward creating a sanctuary that not only feels like home but also bends to their shifting view of the world. It's about giving them a haven that's safe, comforting, and, above all, uncomplicated (*10 Ways to Make Your Home Dementia Friendly*, n.d.).

Easy Eating & Drinking Tips

When it comes to meals and drinks, organization is key. Your loved one's frequently used items should always be within easy reach and kept in consistent, familiar locations.

Involve them in the process of organization, especially when they first move in. **Ask them where they'd like their personal items to be placed**. This fosters a sense of ownership and makes it easier for you to locate these items when they can't remember where they are.

Color contrast can be a powerful tool in a dementia-friendly kitchen. **Equip the kitchen with brightly colored, pattern-free items, from dish towels and plates to glasses.** Everything should contrast with surfaces, walls, and appliances. This makes every item stand out and easy to identify.

In the early stages of dementia, your loved one may still be able to use **basic appliances**. Make sure these **are easily distinguishable and always kept in the same place**.

Food presentation is equally important. **Ensure utensils contrast with both the food and tablecloth**, aiding visibility and reducing confusion.

And finally, remember that clarity is key. **Keep the table free from clutter**, maintaining a clean, organized space that reduces sensory overload and facilitates an enjoyable eating experience.

Bathroom Necessities

Bathroom safety and accessibility are paramount for your loved one. It is crucial that they can easily locate and use the bathroom. Aim for contrast: The **toilet seat and lid should stand out from the rest of the toilet**.

To ensure stability, **add handrails**—vital support for them to steady themselves. These should be fitted not just near the toilet but also in the shower area, helping with balance and assisting them as they step in and out of the bath or shower.

Clearly **mark taps with 'hot' and 'cold' signs** to avoid confusion. Remember, the overarching aim is to create a safe environment that minimizes the risk of slips and falls. This includes **placing non-slip mats in the shower and bath** and **installing flood-prevention**

plugs in your basins and tubs. These handy devices ensure excess water is released down the drain if a tap is inadvertently left running.

Given the vulnerability of dementia sufferers, the risk of scalding is a serious concern. Counteract this by **installing thermostatic mixing valves**. These clever devices automatically blend hot water with cold, ensuring a consistently safe, warm temperature.

Bathing can be a delicate task, requiring a balance between providing necessary supervision and respecting their privacy. Strive to **honor their dignity** during these personal moments.

Keep the bathroom **tidy and uncluttered**, with only essential items in clear sight. **Aim for color contrast**—even toilet paper and towels should stand out from the walls and floors. To help your loved one locate the facilities, **put a sign (preferably pictorial) on the toilet and bathroom doors**. You might also consider leaving these doors open, with lights on during the night for easier navigation.

Finally, it may be best to **remove any bins or trash cans** from these spaces as they could potentially be mistaken for the toilet.

Maintaining Continuity: Clear Labels & Familiar Objects

In every room where your loved one normally spends time, **prominently display vital information**: your address, your loved one's name, and emergency contact numbers. This way, essential details are always within easy reach. If you place a telephone in their room, ensure this information is clearly displayed nearby.

Consistency is key for dementia sufferers. **Always keep their important belongings in the same place**—this can help maintain a sense of continuity and familiarity.

Help your loved one navigate their surroundings by **labeling your cupboards and drawers, indicating their contents**. Opt for pictorial labels where possible, as visual cues can often be more easily understood.

For cupboards, **consider doors that are transparent, nonreflective, and shatterproof**. This lets your loved one see the contents without needing to open the door and minimizes potential confusion or accidents.

Finally, make sure to **leave all room doors wide open**. This will allow your loved one to move easily and unhindered throughout the house, making their day-to-day life much easier (Alzheimer's Society, n.d.).

Promoting Safety: A Protected Environment

Creating a safe haven for someone with Alzheimer's involves tailoring your home to their evolving needs and ensuring that every corner is secure. Here's a guide to turning your home into a fortress of safety, making sure your loved one can navigate their surroundings with ease and confidence:

- **Fire Safety Essentials**: Install fire extinguishers and smoke detectors in key locations. Example: Place a smoke detector in the kitchen and near bedrooms to catch any signs of smoke before they become a bigger issue.
- **Secure Hazardous Areas**: Use child-proof locks and covers on doors and drawers that hold dangerous items. Example: Install a child-proof lock on the cabinet containing cleaning supplies to prevent accidental poisonings.
- **Controlled Access**: Restrict entry to risky areas like the tool shed or kitchen by locking doors or using disguised covers. Example: Fit a disguised panel over the workshop door to prevent wandering into potentially dangerous tools.
- **Bathroom Safety**: Fix grab bars next to the toilet, in the shower, and near the bathtub to help with safe movement.
- **Furniture Familiarity**: Keep the furniture layout consistent once your loved one has adapted to it. Once you find a furniture arrangement that works, keep it that way to avoid confusion and potential falls.
- **Safe Seating**: Ensure chairs have sturdy armrests to support getting up and sitting down. Choose a recliner with long, strong armrests that provide leverage when standing up.
- **Softened Edges**: Pad sharp furniture edges and attach corner guards to the edges of counters and coffee tables to prevent injuries.
- **Pipe Protection**: Insulate exposed hot-water pipes to prevent burns. Example: Wrap foam padding around the pipes under the kitchen and bathroom sinks.
- **Electrical Safety**: Use child-proof plugs on all unused electrical outlets—especially at levels within easy reach.
- **Lock Down**: Keep areas like the garage or basement locked and keep remote controls out of sight. Example: Use a keypad lock for the garage door and keep the opener in a locked drawer.
- **Secure Exits**: Install safety latches and alarms on doors leading outside. Example: Fit an alarm that sounds when the back door is opened.
- **Key Control**: Store all important keys in a secure spot out of reach. Example: Keep car and house keys in a combination lockbox.

Minimizing Fall Risks

Non-slip Solutions: Apply non-slip decals to bath and shower floors. Use textured stickers on bathroom tiles to prevent slipping after a shower.

Declutter and Streamline: Keep walking paths clear of unnecessary furniture and clutter. Regularly check hallways and living spaces to remove anything that could cause a trip.

Furniture Placement: Arrange furniture to accommodate mobility aids like walkers or wheelchairs, ensuring ample space to maneuver. Set the living room furniture against the walls to create clear pathways.

Stable Furniture: Secure furniture so it doesn't shift when leaned on. Place non-slip pads under the legs of the sofa and chairs.

Trip-free Living: Keep the home free from any tripping hazards like loose rugs or electrical cords across walkways. Tape down or remove small area rugs and ensure cords are bundled and off the floor.

Door Safety: Adjust doors to close slowly or remove doors that snap shut quickly. Example: Install slow-close hinges on doors to prevent them from slamming.

Enlist the expertise of caregiving professionals to conduct a home safety evaluation, providing personalized recommendations to further enhance the safety of your living space. Companies like Home Instead offer these assessments as part of their service, ensuring every aspect of your home is optimized for dementia care. (*Home Safety for Families Living With Alzheimer's*, n.d.)

Home Instead website

By taking these proactive steps, you create a living environment that not only supports the specific needs of your loved one with Alzheimer's but also provides peace of mind, knowing that they are safe and secure in their own home.

Wandering—A Prevailing Risk & Some Precautions

Earlier in this chapter, we shared the story of Joe's mom, who, while under his care, began to wander in a state of confusion and daze after he momentarily got distracted by a phone call. This example underscores the swift nature of wandering behaviors common among those living with dementia. Unfortunately, such scenarios happen all too frequently, hence the critical importance of ensuring safety within your home.

Wandering is a daunting reality—more than 60% of dementia sufferers tend to wander away from the safety of their homes. It's of utmost importance, therefore, to adapt your living space in a manner that discourages unattended wandering by your loved one. Experts suggest that fear, confusion, delusions, or hallucinations can trigger such wandering. For instance, they might suddenly believe they're late for work and impulsively walk out, or they may wander in search of their former home or even a bathroom (*Wandering*, n.d.). So, how can you help mitigate this issue? Here are some practical measures:

Install Out-of-Sight Deadbolts: Place deadbolts high or low on exterior doors to deter wandering. For instance, a deadbolt at the top of the door can be out of direct line of sight and reach.

Illuminate Pathways with Night Lights: Strategically place night lights in hallways and bathrooms to guide nighttime movements.

Disguise Doorknobs: Cover knobs with fabric matching the door color, or use child-safety covers, making them less noticeable and reducing the urge to venture outside.

Camouflage Exit Doors: Paint doors the same color as the walls or use curtains to make them blend in, lessening their prominence.

Create Visual Barriers: Use black tape or paint to make a 'stop' line in front of doors, acting as a visual cue not to cross.

Signal Door Usage: Install bells or alarms on doors to alert you when they are opened.

Use Movement Alerts: Place pressure-sensitive mats at doorways to notify you of movement.

Secure Outdoor Spaces: Encircle patios with hedges or fencing to safely confine outdoor areas without feeling restricted.

Install Safety Gates: Use gates or netting to block off stairs and limit outdoor access, ensuring safe movement within the home.

Manage Noise Levels: Keep the home environment calm, as excessive noise can confuse and overwhelm.

Design Safe Exploration Zones: Arrange indoor and outdoor common areas that encourage safe exploration and movement.

Label Doors Clearly: Use signs or symbols to clearly mark what each room is for, aiding in orientation.

Control Triggers: Keep items that might prompt leaving, like coats or keys, out of sight to avoid spontaneous exits.

Never Leave Them Alone in a Car: This can prevent both confusion and potential danger.

Be Prepared: Emergency Planning

Enroll in a Response Service: Consider a service specifically for individuals who may wander, significantly reducing response times if they get lost.

Inform Your Community: Ask neighbors and friends to watch for unusual behavior and alert you immediately if they spot it.

Keep Identification Handy: Have a current photo and important medical information easily accessible to aid in searches.

Familiarize Yourself with the Area: Know the neighborhood and pinpoint hazardous spots that might attract or endanger your loved one.

Compile a List of Likely Places: Note locations your loved one might try to visit, like previous homes or favorite spots, to check during searches.

Immediate Actions for Wandering Incidents

Act Quickly: Start searching immediately, as those who wander are often found close to home.

Check Familiar Spots: Look in areas where they've been found before or might be drawn to due to past routines.

Inform Authorities Promptly: If not found within 15 minutes, contact emergency services and provide them with all necessary information about your loved one's condition and possible destinations.

Remember, understanding and accommodating the needs of your loved one living with dementia is a vital part of their care. Your patience, attentiveness, and flexibility are crucial in fostering a secure and nurturing environment for them.

As we turn to the next chapter, we'll dive deep into the experiences of fellow caregivers. This section is filled with collective wisdom, practical advice, and heartfelt insights, carefully gathered to support you through the complex middle and late stages of dementia care.

Chapter 6: The Mid-Stage Maze

> "Each sunrise brings an opportunity to start anew, even amidst the roughest of tides. And your boundless capacity to love will forever guide and illuminate the path for those entrusted to your care." —S.R. Hatton

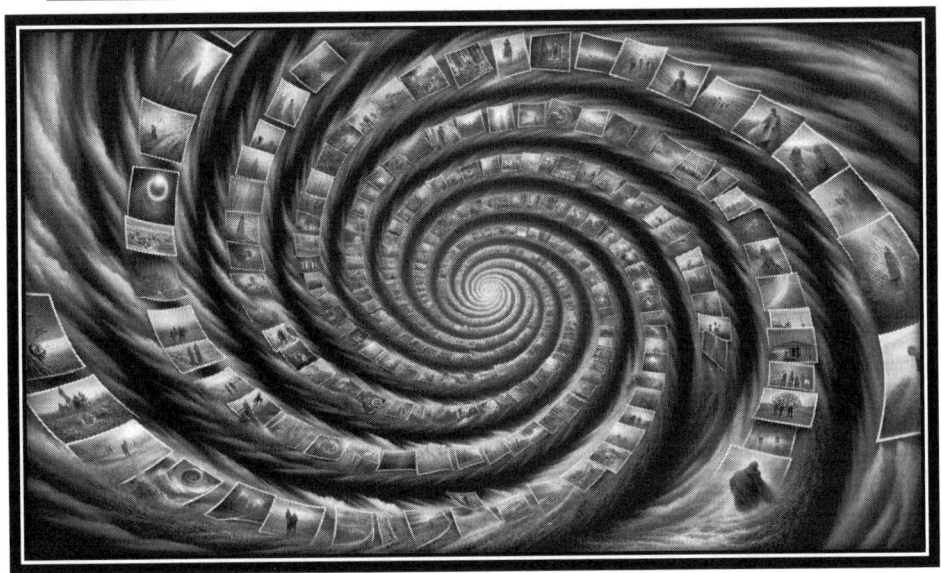

Thriving Through the Challenges of Middle-Stage Dementia

Venturing into the heart of the dementia journey, we meet the longest stretch: the middle stage. The Social Care Institute offers an unvarnished portrayal of this period, which usually lasts for about two to four years but can span over a decade. As your loved one's memory fades, you'll bear witness to their struggles, accompany them through the maze of confusion, and hold their hand as the fog of forgetting thickens.

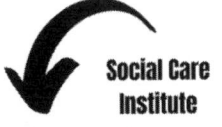

Bear in mind, however, that dementia does not completely obliterate self-awareness. Moments of anger, confusion, and forgetfulness do not mean they have lost all understanding of their circumstances. Just as you feel the heartache watching their transformation, so do they grapple with the bewilderment of their shifting reality. Can you imagine the frustration of not understanding why they were crying earlier or finding themselves inexplicably on the rooftop?

As a caregiver, your strength and resilience will be tested during this period. Some may feel the need to pause their own lives, but let me reassure you—it's not mandatory. With careful balance and some adaptation, you can continue to chase your dreams and maybe even uncover new passions. After all, this journey with your loved one will reshape you, perhaps in ways you never anticipated.

The Social Care Institute conducted interviews with dementia sufferers in a bid to shed light on their experiences, producing a revealing documentary. You might find it surprising when a dementia sufferer of 15 years still recognizes his past self and life, but cannot recall the location of everyday items like tea, sugar, or jam in his kitchen.

Remember this—your loved one is still there, somewhere behind the veil of dementia. They are still capable of insight, of feeling, of existing in their own unique way. The journey into the middle stage may be difficult, but they still harbor a wealth of understanding within them.

By gaining a deeper understanding of their experiences, we can better support our loved ones. As the documentary emphasizes, families and caregivers provide a vital lifeline, helping them navigate their changing world with grace and dignity. You, too, can provide this for your loved one.

Barry

Living with dementia for over 15 years, he remains an articulate speaker, painting vivid pictures of his experiences, sentiments, and perspectives. By sharing his journey, he invites those around him to witness the world through his eyes, grasping the profound challenges he encounters daily. As captured by the Social Care Institute, his words weave an intimate narrative of a life intertwined with dementia ([Social Care Institute for Excellence](#) (SCIE), 2014):

> *"I wake up and feel afraid to get out of bed. I have this fear about what I am going to face today and what may go wrong. I always have this thing in my mind: a feeling that I have done something wrong. Maybe I have broken something. Maybe I have lost something. This thought often comes up for me, 'You aren't good to anybody anymore.' I feel defeated. I just sit here now and do nothing. I am fed and washed. I sleep a lot more. I live like an animal.*
>
> *When I went out last night and came back, my wife offered me a cup of tea upon my return. So, I said, 'That's alright, I'll make the tea.' But I forget where things were kept in the cupboard. I didn't know where to find things*

anymore. I didn't even know if that was my kitchen. Here I am, living with dementia, not knowing where the jam and tea bags are kept.

I used to run a care home before getting dementia. I also managed butcher shops in my life. Now I can't find the sugar, tea, or jam. Dementia stole my life. I didn't see it coming—this sickness. It attacked my mind. It's like a spy. Someone who is not recognizable. But I am a man. I am still me. I have a wife, and my son's dead. People go like, 'Oh, he's got dementia!' Full stop. 'He's senile now!' That is not all that I am. There's still more to me than getting dementia and being forgetful."

Olive

Now residing in a care home for the past two years, Olive's life has taken a profound turn. Her narrative unfolds under the same watchful eyes of the interviewers from the Social Care Institute. Here's how Olive articulates her experiences living with this condition (Social Care Institute for Excellence (SCIE), 2014):

"It's awful. You're hurting the people you love the most. I just don't want to talk to anyone anymore. I know that I am going to repeat myself. So, I don't like talking to anyone. It doesn't feel as if you're in the world anymore. I don't feel like I am part of the world anymore. My family is very caring. I get big hugs from my husband and my children, and they often say, 'That's alright, Mom. You forgot something, that's all.'"

Judy

Diagnosed with dementia in 2004, Judy finds herself on a twisting path of visual perceptual issues, frequently finding herself lost amidst a fog of confusion and disorientation. Despite these challenges, she bravely faces each day, sharing her unique perspective with the interviewers. However, even in the midst of these exchanges, her confusion surfaces, painting a heart-rending portrait of her journey through dementia (Social Care Institute for Excellence (SCIE), 2014):

"I just couldn't go outside anymore. I can't go to a shop or something. I think I'd die if I went outside or something. I used to have fun. Let me live. Where am I? I know who I am. I got that one down. What place is this place? It's still me; it's still me with dementia. I am still me."

Bob

Within the secure confines of a care home for the past two years, Bob carries the unseen burden of dementia. His mind is a theater of vivid hallucinations that come to life daily, so real that they blur the lines between reality and imagination. He finds himself ensnared in webs of mistaken beliefs that fuel these mental spectacles. One memorable instance painted his room with imaginary flames, causing him to flee from the perceived danger. Even more shocking, before his transition to the care home, he found himself twice atop his house, a chilling testament to the disorienting power of his condition ([Social Care Institute for Excellence](#) (SCIE), 2014).

> *"I got up and walked across the roof of the house. I don't know what made me do it. I can't explain it. All I can say is that it happened, and I did it. It happened at one am in the morning. That is quite frightening. I used to be doing great at one time. But every year now, it just gets harder and harder. I have trouble concentrating. I just can't concentrate anymore on anything. My mind goes blank. I don't think you realize how it hits you. It's a silent illness. It creeps up on you. I feel lonely. Dementia makes me lonely. I didn't see that coming."*

What to Anticipate in the Middle Stages

The complex web of communication: As dementia's grip tightens, expressing thoughts and feelings becomes an intricate puzzle, their words morphing into a jumbled cacophony.

Dressing up—a towering hurdle: They will grapple with this mundane task, triggering bouts of anger and frustration.

The growing rebellion: There may be vehement refusals to bathe or comply with other routine aspects.

The fading patchwork of memory: Expect memory and thinking patterns to take a hit, transforming familiar faces into strangers and stretching the time it takes to process and remember new information.

Echoes in conversation: Repetition will become a constant companion as they start to reiterate themselves more frequently.

The challenge of concentration: Attention span dwindles, making it harder for them to follow your conversations or maintain focus.

The encroaching shadow of depression: Middle stages of dementia often bring in this uninvited guest, adding a layer of melancholy to their emotional state.

The distortion of reality: False beliefs, delusions, and hallucinations may take root, leading them to level accusations of unfaithfulness at their partners or perceive nonexistent sights and sounds.

Raising the volume: Expect an increase in screaming and shouting as frustration and confusion mount.

The shadow of suspicion: They might start tailing you, fueled by the suspicion that you might be plotting against them.

Shedding inhibitions: Embarrassing actions may unfold in public as they lose their inhibitions, which may include spontaneous undressing.

Sleep, an elusive visitor: Disturbed sleeping patterns will become the norm.

The (non)independence of toileting: Using the toilet on their own might turn into a challenging feat.

The transition from the early to the middle stages of dementia is like crossing a rapidly moving river; it's more intense and can feel sudden. The waves might seem overwhelming, but remember that you are not alone. Arm yourself with the right resources and embrace the evolving relationship with your loved one. The upcoming challenges may seem daunting, but every hurdle you overcome will teach you invaluable lessons and strategies shared by healthcare professionals (*The Middle Stage of Dementia*, 2021). Every day is a new chance to learn and grow stronger together.

Real-World Tips & Tricks for Middle-Stage Dementia

Now, let's get more specific around communication:

> *"In your conversations, treat them like you would any other person. Discuss the weather, their pets, or compliment their appearance. Yet, be ready to master the art of distraction and deflection. Each day may bring different levels of communication skills and memory abilities. One day, they may seem perfectly lucid, as if dementia has temporarily loosened its grip. On another day, they may weave fantastical stories, accusing you of stealing their favorite sweater under the cover of night. Their reality can fluidly move between recognizing you and viewing you as a high school classmate.*
>
> *Your tool here is to gently steer the conversation. 'Indeed, our math teacher was stern, wasn't he? How about a glass of water or a stroll in the garden?' It's vital to align yourself with their reality rather than pulling them out of it, unless it puts them in harm's way. If they're having a conversation with an unseen entity who, in actuality, passed away a decade ago, don't abruptly remind them of their loss. Every reminder is a fresh wound, a reawakening of old grief. Accept their reality as they present it—if they offer you an imaginary cup of coffee, simply say thank you.*
>
> *The journey of dementia, as your loved one progressively declines, is a challenge navigated best with gentleness and patience. Stress and anxiety can intensify their symptoms, potentially elevate blood pressure and, in some cases, lead to mini-strokes in patients with vascular dementia. Your goal is to reduce confusion and create a calm, comforting environment. It's about sailing along with their currents, rather than resisting them, ensuring a smoother journey through the turbulent waters of dementia."* —Anonymous Quora Contributor

> *"As a healthcare professional, I've learned to embrace their conversations, no matter how nonsensical they may seem to me. If you're trying to persuade them to do something, such as wearing clean clothes, eating, or bathing, it's important to communicate in a way that resonates with their current reality. You might say something like, 'Mom told us we must put on clean clothes for school,' as an example. Avoid confrontation or forcing*

them to act against their will. They live in their own unique world, and unless it poses a threat to their safety or the safety of others, it's best to allow them to enjoy it. Remember, your role isn't to correct their perception of reality, but rather to make their journey through it as peaceful and enjoyable as possible." —Quora Contributor

"As a valuable piece of advice for those communicating with someone living with Alzheimer's who's largely lost verbal expression, consider the creation of visual aids. Flashcards or cut-out images from magazines, or even printed ones from a computer, could represent their usual requests. This could include a 'toilet,' a 'drink,' or a depiction of feelings such as 'pain,' 'hot,' or 'cold.' Arrange the most frequently used images on a piece of cardboard covered with clear contact paper for longevity. This way, they can point to what they need or feel. If they still possess the ability to write, a dry-erase board can also be a handy tool. This visual communication strategy can alleviate frustration and provide them with a valuable means of expressing their needs and feelings." —Facebook Group contributors

In the complex journey of dementia care, you may find yourself facing a paradoxical choice: the need to lie to them. Yes, you heard me right: **You may need to lie to them**. It sounds counterintuitive, doesn't it? We're raised to value honesty, but in the realm of dementia, reality can sometimes be too harsh for your loved one to process.

Engaging in what's known as 'therapeutic fibbing' can become a necessary part of communication as dementia progresses. This approach isn't about deceiving for personal gain but about protecting your loved one from distress. The art of this practice requires a delicate balance of compassion and pragmatism, guided by the intention to soothe rather than deceive.

As you adapt to this aspect of caregiving, let the shared experiences of others in similar situations be your guide. Many caregivers have walked this path before you, employing empathy and kindness when straightforward facts would do more harm than good.

"During the initial transition into a new care facility, my mother constantly yearned for her beloved home, the one she'd lived in and cherished for over two decades. At the same time, I found myself bearing the tough responsibility of emptying out that apartment and selling the car she had

meticulously chosen just a few years prior. Driven by the necessity of her care expenses, I did what I had to do.

I began to adopt a comforting narrative that I would repeat to her: 'Mom, according to your doctor, it's crucial that you stay here until you regain your health. Please remember to take your medication, engage in your exercises, and you'll be back home before you know it!' This was my iteration of the truth, always with a sliver of hope that a miracle might reverse the course of her dementia.

Once I adjusted to the ever-changing levels of her cognition, I understood that small white lies were necessary for her peace of mind. Whether it was news of her best friend and brother's passing or her sister's recent dementia diagnosis, I gently framed the truth to preserve her sense of security and happiness. Even the sale of her car was woven into a tale where she would be able to drive again as soon as the doctor approved.

Witnessing her joy as she clutched her expired license and a few dollars in her purse made it all worthwhile. When she would mention my deceased father or her mother, I learned to play along, reassuring her that 'I'm sure they'll come by to visit soon.'

There may be times when the 'sundowning' phenomenon takes hold, generating strong negative illusions. I once cared for a woman who was convinced that bugs were creeping out of her kitchen sink. It's important to understand that denying their perceived reality only adds to their stress. Instead, assure them that the problem has been resolved and will never recur. And if they've adopted any unconventional coping mechanisms, try to gently steer them towards a safer alternative.

Adopting these approaches doesn't mean that you're being dishonest. Instead, you're offering your loved ones a refuge in their own reality, ensuring they feel comforted and reassured in the world they're navigating." — Unknown Quora contributor

Navigating through the delicate matters of life, loss, and memory in the world of dementia care is akin to walking a tightrope. It's a delicate balance of truth, compassion, and preservation of peace. Here's an enlightening encounter from my own experience that might offer you a better perspective on this intricate dance.

My beloved Grandma Bonnie had been a resident at the care facility for a considerable length of time, and her husband of 55 years (my sweet Grandpa 'Bud') was her constant companion, visiting her faithfully. However, the day arrived when he passed away, leaving us in a dilemma about how, or even **if**, we should share this heartbreaking news with her.

During a family visit to the facility, we made the tough decision to reveal that her devoted husband no longer walked among us. As anticipated, the news was a blow to her heart. She reacted with disbelief, shock, and sorrow, shedding tears that shook us to our core. The room was awash with grief, and even the staff scrambled to find enough tissues to dry our collective tears.

But, as our sobs ebbed away, Grandma Bonnie looked up, her tear-stained face wearing a question. She asked, "Has anyone seen Bud this morning?" The confusion and concern on my mother's and aunt's faces were palpable. They dreaded the thought of their mother reliving that pain all over again.

However, with barely a second's hesitation, my aunt responded with an incredible wisdom I've since recognized as the most compassionate response one could offer in such a situation. She softly told her, "He's resting, Momma." (Which, in essence, wasn't **that** far from the truth.) To this, Grandma Bonnie replied, "Oh, okay. He **was** pretty tired when he got up this morning."

From then on, every time she asked about her husband, she would be told this gentle untruth, which she readily accepted. The beauty of it was that she never had to suffer the anguish of losing him ever again.

The hard truth of the matter is simply this: Sometimes, in the world of dementia care, a little white lie can be like giving your loved one a comfort blanket instead of a cold splash of reality. It's all about preserving their peace and emotional well-being.

Now, let's get into some tips around dressing and bathing:

"<u>No one dies of stink</u>; there's always a work-around. Use bird baths instead of full-blown showers or baths in a tub—less sensory stimulation, less anxiety. Fill the sink with warm water, get some pleasantly scented soap-stuff (not a lot of soap; soap dries skin, and an itchy person with dementia won't be fun to be around. Better the smell of body odor), a washcloth, and have the person wash themselves [if they are able]—face, underarms, genitals. A full-on shower or bath isn't necessary, and the stress of forcing a person with dementia to do something which distresses them so much is a recipe for a catastrophic reaction." —Anonymous Quora contributor

"<u>Much of the refusing care is common</u>. As they progress through stages of dementia, especially mid and early late stages, they seem aware of a loss of control of their lives as more and more people, often strangers to them, are doing things for them (A loss of independence frustrates them. Refusing care, even refusing to eat, is their way of trying to gain back control, gain back independence.)

It's not a quick fix but it may help to add choices to their everyday lives. Keep the choices simple and keep to a routine. Keep choices to 2. This shirt or that shirt? Rice or pasta? Play cards or build birdhouses?

When it comes to bathing, don't ask 'yes bath or no bath,' say, 'It's Friday. Do you want to bathe first or shave first?' If they balk after that, go with choice again, 'The blue soap or the yellow soap?' Notice, again, that not bathing isn't one of the choices.

Keep in mind that many people of their generation bathed instead of showered. Is there any way you can retro fit the shower into a sitting tub with a shower head for rinsing off?

People with dementia forget much of what occurs fairly quickly, but they do remember feelings. They may not remember the last time they bathed but they will remember that they felt forced or angry or scared about bathing.

With my own mother (she is physically capable of bathing but can't remember how to fill or drain the tub or to remember to bathe), I run her a very warm (not hot, never hot) bath with LOTS of lavender bubble bath. I

unhook the shower head so it hangs where she can reach it. After she bathes, I remind her how to trigger the shower portion, and she sprays herself off. It's taken several weeks but she's much more amenable to bathing when I ask her to now. I finally figured out WHY she didn't bathe. Turned out she couldn't figure out the faucet and her previous baths were cold. She hated bathing in cold water, so she hated bathing." —A Certified Dementia Practitioner, answering a question on Quora.com

Adaptive Bras on Amazon

"<u>The only time mom takes her bra off is to shower</u>. She lives with my husband and I and is not allowed to go braless. If not going anywhere, we let her stay in her pajamas or sweat clothes. At times, mom sleeps in her sweats. Also, there are things called '<u>adaptive bras</u>' for elderly women or women with arthritis [which can be found on Amazon]. They can sleep in them and are much easier to get on and off than regular bras." —Anonymous Facebook Group member

"<u>My MIL struggles with pulling her pants up & down</u> to use the bathroom and getting dressed/undressed. So, we bought her a few of those 'moo-moo' dresses to wear around the house. It seems to have helped the situation some. Though at times she likes to pull up the dress and show her underwear. Some of the staff at the MC facility also suggested we get her some of those stretchy jumpsuits since they are comfortable and easier to get on and off." — Anonymous Facebook Group member

In the complex network of the human mind, dementia is a cruel saboteur. Its insidious presence has the power to drastically alter an individual's demeanor, conjuring up bouts of aggression and volatile behavior in its wake. It's a battle they never chose to fight, yet it's unfolding inside their brain, beyond their control or consent. Research from the National Institutes of Health showed that up to 96 percent of patients with dementia studied over 10 years showed aggressive behavior at some point (Jackson & Mallory, 2009). But amidst the storm, there is hope. The following real-world tips and tricks will unveil some practical strategies, accumulated from years of dedicated research and lived experiences, all designed to **help navigate the choppy seas of dementia-induced aggression**.

"Identify the cause: Aggressive behavior could be a reaction to pain, confusion, fear, or frustration. Try to uncover what's triggering these reactions so you can address it effectively.

For example, your LOWD might start yelling at empty areas of the room and telling people to get out. Looking around, you might notice that the room is starting to get darker because it's early evening. The dim light causes shadowing in the corners of the room, making it seem like there are people in the corner.

After identifying that potential trigger, turn on the lights to get rid of the shadowy corners. That will hopefully help your LOWD calm down. And, in the future, you'll know to turn on the lights before the room gets too dim.

In another example, you could have unintentionally approached your loved one from behind and startled them. In a sensitive moment, that could make them feel attacked, so they lash out in what they perceive as self-defense.

Many older adults with dementia aren't able to clearly communicate when something is bothering them. Instead, being in pain or discomfort could cause them to act out. Other common causes of aggression in dementia patients are dehydration and urinary tract infections.

Be sure to check to see if they need pain medication for existing conditions like arthritis or gout, if their seat is comfortable, or if they need to use the toilet.

Stay calm: Maintaining a calm and patient demeanor is vital. Responding with anger could escalate the situation and create more tension.

When your LOWD gets upset, take a deep breath and stay as calm as possible. If you're upset, that unintentionally continues escalating the tense emotions in the situation.

Staying calm and breathing slowly helps to reduce everyone's anger and agitation. Speak slowly and keep your voice soft, reassuring, and positive.

If appropriate, use a gentle and calming touch on the arm or shoulder to provide comfort and reassurance.

Aromatherapy, music therapy, reminiscence, occupational therapy, as well as art activities may be beneficial and have a calming or rewarding effect for the person with dementia.

Use distraction: Changing the subject or activity can often defuse a difficult situation. This approach can redirect the person's attention and ease their aggression.

If the current or previous activity caused agitation or frustration, it could have provoked an aggressive response.

After giving your LOWD a minute to vent their feelings, try to shift their attention to a different activity—something they typically enjoy.

Validate their feelings: It's important to let the person know their feelings are recognized and valid. Phrases like "I understand you're upset, and it's okay to feel this way," can be comforting.

Ensure a safe environment: A calm, quiet environment free from potential anxiety triggers can help lessen agitation and aggressive behavior.

If your LOWD starts behaving aggressively, take notice of the environment to see if you can quickly calm the room. Turn down the music volume, turn off the TV, and ask other people to leave the room.

In some cases, nothing works to calm the person. If that happens, it may be best to leave the room to give them some space and give yourself time to calm down and regain balance. They may be able to calm themselves or might even forget that they're angry.

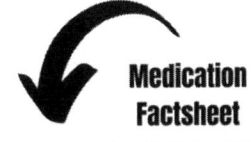

But before leaving, check to see that the environment is safe and that they're not likely to hurt themselves while you're gone.

Consider medication: In some instances, medication might be necessary to manage aggressive behavior." (This factsheet from the Alzheimer's Society has some great information about drug treatments, but be sure to first consult with a healthcare provider to discuss if this is an appropriate option for your LOWD.)

"There are several drugs available today for improving brain function and reducing dementia symptoms. Typically, anti-dementia or other psychotropic drugs are prescribed.

Some types are the **anti-dementia** agents belonging to the so-called acetylcholinesterase inhibitors class of drugs. Acetylcholine is one of the chemical substances that allow brain cells to communicate with one another, the so-called neurotransmitters. Research suggests that acetylcholine is reduced in the brains of AD patients. These kinds of drugs prevent acetylcholine from being eliminated too quickly, prolonging its ability to conduct chemical messages between brain cells. It could be shown in clinical trials that, with these kinds of drugs, the deterioration of the disease could be delayed by at least 12 months. Apart from preserving and partially improving mental capacities, and coping with daily activities, delayed onset of behavioral disturbances and a reduction in caring time could also be demonstrated.

Psychotropic drugs can be used as supportive therapy in the treatment of behavioral problems in dementia. For instance, antipsychotic medications (typically used to treat disorders like schizophrenia) can be effective in reducing persistent aggression in patients who have been unresponsive to non-pharmacological approaches, and where there is a risk of harm to themselves or others; however, such treatments should be used only short-term—up to six weeks—rather than on a systematic basis.

Anti-anxiety medications (typically used to treat anxiety disorders) can also be prescribed to help treat agitation and restlessness. Likewise, antidepressant medication can be prescribed to alleviate symptoms of depression. Treating depression symptoms is particularly important, as depression makes it harder for a person with dementia to remember things and enjoy life. It also adds to the difficulty of caring for someone with dementia. Significant improvements can be made by treating depression, as the patient's mood and ability to participate in activities may be improved.

In general, medications should be administered very cautiously to patients with dementia and in the lowest possible effective doses, to minimize side effects. Supervision of taking medications is generally required. With each of these medications, there are associated side effects and risks. Therefore, a careful risk-benefit evaluation should be conducted before treatment initiation and regularly throughout treatment. However, one must bear in mind that these medications do not cure dementia or reverse someone's symptoms. There is no evidence that life is prolonged by taking medications. Rather, these medications can help some patients function better for a longer period." (For additional information about treatment options, the Alzheimer's Association has several pages on their website dedicated to this.)

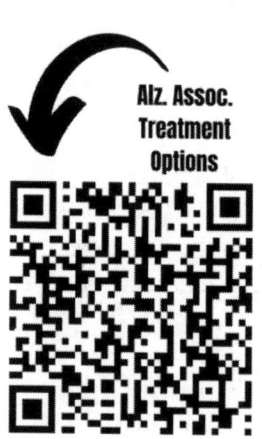

Alz. Assoc. Treatment Options

"Seek support: Don't forget to take care of yourself, too. Reach out to family, friends, and professional caregivers to share the load and ensure you're well-supported.

If you find yourself in a situation where your LOWD can't calm down and is becoming a danger to you or to themselves, you'll need help from others.

If the situation isn't extreme and there's a nearby family member or friend that your loved one usually responds well to, call and ask them to come over to help immediately.

In an emergency, call 911 and emphasize to the operator that the person has dementia, which is causing them to act aggressively. This helps first responders know that the person isn't behaving criminally and needs help to calm down safely.

When first responders arrive, **make sure you again clearly state that this behavior is caused by dementia** or even 'a brain injury' (in case they're not familiar with dementia). That knowledge helps first responders treat them more appropriately.

If your loved one needs to be removed from the home, ask that they be taken to a hospital or psychiatric institution rather than to a police station.

Assuming that you don't want to press charges, make it very clear that this behavior is caused by dementia (or 'mental illness'—might be easier to understand) and not criminal behavior. That helps avoid formal charges or unwanted court proceedings.

Remember, everyone is unique: Each person with dementia responds differently. It might take some time to discover the strategies that work best for the individual you're caring for." —Various Quora Contributors

Some additional (and important) advice around medications for dementia patients was posted by a member of a Dementia Facebook Group:

"Medication is available to help ease anxiety and aggression. Also, to help with hallucinations and delusional behaviors. Keep in mind though that it is not usually an instant fix. Some of these medications require 4-6 weeks to obtain a therapeutic level in the blood and body, depending on the individual. Doses may need to be adjusted as well. In my nursing experience with these issues, I have rarely seen any improvement in the first two weeks. A major mistake, and a dangerous one, is frequently made when the drug doesn't appear to be working as it should the first 2-4 weeks and without doing any lab evaluation the dose is increased. This can cause toxicity to occur and increase the behaviors or damage kidneys. Blood work to ascertain the levels of the medication in the blood should be done every two weeks or whenever symptoms/behaviors seem to worsen for the first 6 weeks of drug therapy. These medications can be beneficial but should be closely monitored."

Envision dementia as an uninvited traveler taking a reverse trip through the milestones of human development. As the journey unfolds, the brain morphs, not towards the wisdom of age, but regresses towards the innocence of infancy. Picture the trajectory: from the complexities of adulthood, the brain winds back to the impulsiveness of adolescence, then to the explorative curiosity of childhood, and ultimately, the helplessness of an infant. This downward spiral results in the person forgetting even the most fundamental human functions. They may lose understanding of what a toilet represents, become incapable of deciphering bodily cues related to bladder or bowel movements, and lack the control to regulate the muscles governing waste expulsion. It's crucial to grasp this grim reality to foster empathy and provide effective care, realizing that the afflicted individual has no control over this horrible transformation.

According to an article in Healthline.com, one hurdle that often emerges in the journey through dementia is urinary incontinence—an unintentional loss of bladder control that can manifest anywhere from minor leakage to full-blown uncontrolled urination. In some cases, it can also extend to fecal incontinence, translating to unintentional bowel movements, from occasional stool leakage to complete loss of bowel control.

This unsettling symptom typically appears in the latter stages of dementia, affecting approximately 60 to 70 percent of individuals living with dementia. However, it's crucial to understand that this isn't a ubiquitous trait for everyone with dementia—not everyone affected will necessarily encounter this issue (Morris, 2023).

As caregivers, the importance of understanding and managing incontinence can't be overstated. So let's delve into why this occurs, how it interacts with dementia, and arm ourselves with effective management strategies. Knowledge is your best ally here, equipping you to provide the best care and maintain dignity for your loved one, even in the face of these challenging symptoms.

In the later stages of dementia, a person's ability to react quickly and remember things is reduced. They may no longer recognize when they experience the urge to urinate or have a bowel movement. Reasons for incontinence in someone with dementia include:

- not recognizing the bathroom
- communication issues
- being unable to get to the bathroom in time
- mobility loss

In some cases, accidents can lead to feelings of embarrassment and possibly depression.

Certain factors can also increase a person's risk for incontinence. These factors include:
- being overweight, as weight puts pressure on the bladder
- age, as older adults tend to have weaker bladder muscles
- pregnancy and childbirth, which can affect the pelvic floor and bladder muscles
- menopause, as hormones affect the bladder
- enlarged prostate or prostate surgery
- certain medications
- trauma that affects the nerves

Urinary tract infection (UTI) is also common in people with dementia. Watch for signs of UTI, including:
- burning or painful urination
- cloudy or blood-tinged urine
- constant urge to urinate
- pain in the pelvis or back
- fever, nausea, vomiting
- mental status changes or abrupt worsening of confusion, including significant changes in behavior

UTIs can worsen without proper treatment.

Medications are available to calm an overactive bladder if an overactive bladder is the cause of the incontinence. However, some have side effects that can make dementia worse. Talk with the doctor about options that apply to the person you're caring for. In some cases, where incontinence is caused by an underlying medical condition, treating the condition may help.

When managing someone's diet, make sure they:
- avoid carbonation or caffeine
- limit liquids before bed
- avoid spicy or acidic foods, which irritate the urinary tract
- eat plenty of fiber to avoid constipation
- exercise (in some form) regularly

Fluid intake is also important, as it keeps the bladder and bowel healthy. Space out roughly six to eight glasses each day. Fiber-rich foods like bran, fruit, and vegetables can help with constipation.

If the person you're caring for needs to wear absorbent products such as pads, adult underwear, or liners, you may also need to wash their skin. Regular exposure to moisture can cause a number of skin problems, such as inflammation, and fungal and yeast infections.

Keep skin clean by washing it gently with a pH-balanced perineal cleanser and then patting it dry. Creams and powders can be useful in protecting skin from moisture overexposure.

Incontinence often happens due to timing. It may help to recognize potential signs that a person needs to go, such as straining, turning red in the face, and tugging at their clothing. If you help them get dressed, use clothing that's easy to remove, such as pants with elastic waistbands instead of buttons and belts.

One successful technique is prompted voiding. This is a type of bladder retraining that helps people to maintain a regular bathroom schedule. For example, every two hours, ask if they've had an accident, have the person use the toilet, and praise successes.

The goal to reduce accidents at home is to help the person you're caring for identify and use the toilet with ease. Here are some things you can do to achieve this goal:

- Remove obstacles from paths taken most often to the toilet.
- Leave the bathroom door open at all times or put a sign in front of the door. Avoid locking the door.
- Make sure the toilet is at a good height and that lighting is good. Install grab bars next to the toilet, if possible.
- Wait until they are next to the toilet to help remove their clothing.

At night, you can place a portable toilet chair near their bed. Installing motion sensor lights may also help avoid accidents. If they can't get to the bathroom without help, consider getting a bed pad or a waterproof mattress protector (Morris, 2023).

"Dementia's journey isn't one for the faint-hearted; it's full of surprising twists and turns. A challenging milestone that practically every person with dementia will encounter is both urinary and fecal incontinence. To navigate this, arm yourself with the essential tools of the trade: adult diapers, wipes, washcloths, protective creams against chafing, and possibly even a portable toilet. Preparation is paramount.

As a caregiver, it's crucial to be proactive. That means guiding your loved one to the restroom often, as memory loss will rob them of familiar routines—like locating the restroom, using the facilities, and maintaining personal hygiene. Yes, you read it right—diaper changes are on the agenda, too.

In certain scenarios, dementia can lead to unpredictable behavior—from roaming around and pooping or peeing in inappropriate places to interacting with their feces. Brace yourself for these possibilities, they're part of the dementia roller coaster.

If you find this is a ride you can't take, it's absolutely okay. There are professional caregivers and memory care facilities ready to step in. Hiring a home nurse or exploring a nursing home isn't admitting defeat; it's about ensuring the best care for your loved one. So, remember, whatever path you choose, you're doing a remarkable job." — Anonymous Quora contributor

"Adult diapers are the answer when they get to the point where they cannot keep from wetting and soiling their bedding. Maybe find a video showing how to change diapers on a bedridden person." (Yep! I found a great one right here.) "Do you have a turn sheet on top of her fitted sheet to turn her with? If so, turn them on their side and lift their leg up (like a prop) and clean from the back. A turn sheet is a flat sheet folded about 3 times. Giving room for you to reach the sides and then gently pull it toward you and it will turn them more on their side. Helps keep them from getting bed sores, also. You can turn them right or left. Maybe put a rubber-type pad under them as much as possible to keep the sheet clean." —Dementia Facebook Group member

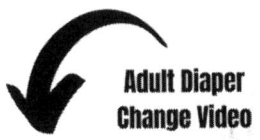

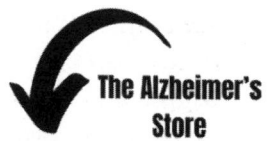

For a loved one who routinely likes to remove their clothing—as well as their Depends or adult diaper—and then proceeds to make a complete mess with the contents of that diaper, a great suggestion from a Dementia Facebook Group member was to buy him/her some "Alzheimer's PJs."

You can shop for these items on Amazon.com or at specialty shops such as The Alzheimer's Store, ProfessionalFit.com, 4Care-USA.com, or Adaptawear.com in the UK.

Now, what about that ever-relentless topic of helping your LOWD use the bathroom—in public? Supporting a loved one with dementia during a public restroom visit requires patience, understanding, and sensitivity, especially when you're of the opposite sex. The first priority is always the comfort and dignity of the person with dementia. Here are a few tips to navigate this scenario:

"*<u>Plan Ahead</u>: Before leaving the house, explain the game plan like a football coach gearing up for the big game—we're taking a trip, and teamwork is crucial. When selecting clothing, imagine it's 'Opposite Day' for a high-security prison. That means no complex locks or confusing contraptions—elastic waistbands and clothes that slide on and off with the elegance of a greased penguin are your friends!*

<u>Scout for Family or Unisex Bathrooms</u>: Upon arrival, launch into detective mode—your mission? Locate the restrooms. A lot of places offer the holy grail: the family or unisex bathroom—the 'Switzerland' of restrooms, neutral territory for all. If this elusive gem is unavailable, you may need to call in backup.

<u>Enlist Help</u>: If faced with the last resort—a gender-segregated restroom—it's time to host your impromptu episode of 'Who Wants to be a Good Samaritan?' Be ready to kindly ask a trustworthy individual of your loved one's sex, or a staff member for assistance. Most folks will be ready for their 15 minutes of fame and happy to help. (Of course, it also depends on whether the business at hand is a Number 1 or a Number 2.)

<u>Narrate the Journey</u>: Keep your loved one in the loop by narrating each step as though you're a radio sportscaster. From opening the door to washing hands afterward, your soothing voice and vivid play-by-play can help reduce their anxiety—and provide them with the exciting restroom commentary they never knew they needed!

<u>Preserve Their Dignity</u>: No matter what, maintaining dignity is essential, so remember you're not their overeager personal assistant. Encourage their independence like a cheerleader on the sidelines—pom-poms optional." —Anonymous Quora Contributor

Remember, every situation will be different, and what works once might not work again. Be patient, flexible, and ready to adapt to the needs of the person with dementia. Providing support in a public restroom may not always be easy, but your compassionate and understanding approach can make a world of difference to the person you're caring for.

There are a plethora of strategies and techniques that can help to make the journey more manageable and less daunting for both you and your loved one. Overall, here are the four key strategies to keep in mind:

1. **Embrace the Role of the Memory Guide:** As dementia burrows its way into the complex network of the brain, it begins to shake the very foundations of reasoning and decision-making, accelerating the pace of memory loss. It's here that you come into play as the memory guide, gently leading the way. Escort them through their tasks, like a tour guide in their own homes, occasionally nudging their memory about the whereabouts of everyday items. When friends come knocking, announce their presence like a herald in the court, ensuring your loved one is aware of the visitor.
2. **Steering through Sundowning:** As the curtain of dusk falls, it often sets off a whirlwind within them—that phenomenon known as sundowning. Reach into your toolkit for the strategies detailed in Chapter 3 to transform these turbulent nights into tranquil ones, anchoring everyone in the harbor of serene slumber.
3. **Encouraging Meaningful Activities:** Like a gardener nurturing vibrant blooms, cultivate an environment of activity and productivity. A bustling mind is like a magician's trick, deftly diverting attention from unsettling hallucinations. Ignite their passions, whether it's immersing them in soothing melodies, encouraging their green thumbs, sparking their inner artist, or rallying behind their favored team on the sports channel.
4. **Building a Robust Support Network:** Caregiving, while rewarding, can also be exhausting. Like the walls of a mighty fortress, having a robust support network provides strength and protection against caregiver burnout. Don't hesitate to lean on friends, family, fellow caregivers, and healthcare professionals when the going gets tough. Seeking help is not an admission of defeat, but rather a brave act of ensuring the best possible care for your loved one.

Handling the care of a loved one with dementia can feel a bit like directing a play where the script changes every scene. As their story unfolds, there might come a time when home care just doesn't cut it anymore, and the spotlight shifts to finding a specialized facility. In this next chapter, we'll tackle the heavyweight decision of when to upgrade to professional care. Pinpointing this crucial switch-up is key to making sure your loved one still gets top-bill treatment.

As someone who was always confused by which type of facility does what, I'm going to explain how to spot the signs that it's time for a change, scout out the most appropriate place for your LOWD, and smooth over the transition. With some strategic directing and a heart full of empathy, you'll be set to guide this shift like a seasoned pro, keeping your loved one's comfort and dignity center stage.

Chapter 7: What To Do When What You Do Just Isn't Enough

"Remove the weight of worry so you may find solace in your grief." —S.R. Hatton

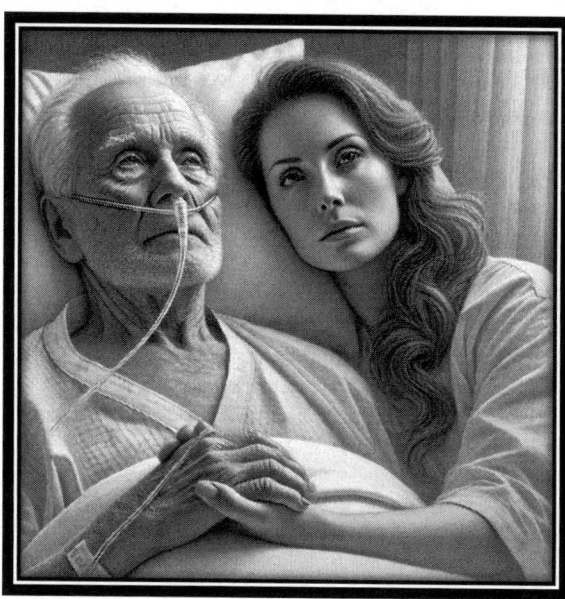

Handling Hospital Hurdles: When Hospitalization Makes Sense

Deciding to hospitalize a loved one with dementia can feel as tricky as deciding whether to restore a vintage car. You're weighing the perks of a tune-up against the potential for causing more dents and scratches. For folks with dementia, a hospital can seem less like a recovery room and more like a haunted house, amping up their confusion and inviting a host of spooky complications like infections or the dreaded delirium.

Start by sizing up the situation. Is this an emergency like severe pain or an infection that demands immediate medical wizardry? If so, hospital time might be non-negotiable. But if we're talking about a bad day with confusion or a sudden bout of crankiness, consider keeping things calm on the home front with treatments that don't involve a hospital bracelet (even a session with the hypnotherapist could do wonders here).

Now, let's get into the nuts and bolts of handling dementia complications. Non-invasive options might keep things smooth, like physical therapy to avoid those pesky falls. However, the heavy-duty fixes—think surgeries or biopsies—need a serious sit-down with the doctor to weigh out the pros and cons.

And don't forget about those advanced directives. These are like your loved one's instruction manual for doctors, making sure their medical care lines up with their personal choices. Have they got a living will? Check it! It's a roadmap for tough calls about life support or other major decisions.

As the head honcho of caregiving, your gig involves more than just nodding along to doctors. You've got to dig deep, ask the hard questions, and sometimes even call foul if the play doesn't suit your loved one's wishes. It's about making sure every medical move is a checkmate for their well-being and dignity.

Comfort First: Introducing Palliative Care for Your LOWD

Palliative care, often misunderstood as solely end-of-life care, is not just the last lap in the healthcare relay; it's a robust strategy to boost comfort and quality of life right from the starting blocks. Far from waving the white flag, this approach rolls out the red carpet for comfort, keeping symptoms in check and ensuring dignity isn't something left on the nightstand.

The trick to maximizing palliative care is timing—think of it like seasoning food; the earlier you add it, the deeper the flavors, or in this case, the better the quality of life. But it's not exclusive to the final stages; it's a good plus-one to have at any point in the dementia journey. Suppose your loved one seems more frazzled than a cat in a yarn store due to symptoms like pain or confusion—it might be time to bring palliative care into the mix. This squad, including doctors, nurses, and social workers, plays well together to ease not just their physical pain, but emotional and spiritual pain, too.

Kicking off palliative care can start with a chat with the doctor—kind of like discussing what's missing in a recipe. Say your dad's getting anxious or agitated. This care style could mix in some calm-inducing meds and relaxing activities to take the edge off. It's all about customizing comfort and making sure your loved one's needs are front and center.

Making sense of palliative choices means mixing a dose of medical insight with a heavy pour of personal preference. Get into the nitty-gritty of what matters most to them. Is being at home a top priority? Any medical moves they want to sidestep? Setting up a game plan that respects these wishes means their care stays as true to them as their favorite old hat—and documenting these details in an advance care plan helps keep everyone in the loop, steering the care ship smoothly as waters get choppy.

Finding resources and support for palliative care can sometimes feel overwhelming. However, many hospitals and clinics now have palliative care teams, and your primary care doctor can often provide a referral. Additionally, organizations like the National Hospice and Palliative Care Organization (NHPCO) offer directories of services and a wealth of information about palliative care and how to access it. (One of their programs, CaringInfo.org, provides specific information about things like the difference between palliative care and hospice care.) Support groups, both in-person and online, can also provide insights and advice from other caregivers who have gone down similar paths, offering both practical tips and emotional support.

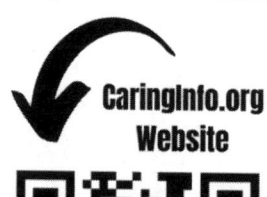

Remember, **palliative care is about adding life to days, not merely days to life**. It's a special form of care that brings comfort, dignity, and tranquility to patients and their families, making the dementia journey as gentle as possible. By understanding its principles, knowing when to integrate it, making informed decisions about care, and utilizing available resources, you ensure that your loved one receives the best possible support, tailored to their needs and respectful of their wishes.

I know that working your way through the maze of medical facilities for your loved one can feel overwhelming, but understanding the distinct types of care available can illuminate the best path for your LOWD. Whether you're looking for a place that balances independence with support, a specialized environment for dementia care, or comprehensive medical supervision, each type of facility offers unique advantages tailored to specific needs. In this section, we'll explore assisted living facilities, memory care units, and what many people refer to as 'nursing homes,' delving into the nuances of each to help you make informed decisions about the best care options for your LOWD.

Assisted Living Facilities: These are designed for seniors who need some help with daily activities such as bathing, dressing, and medication management but do not require constant medical care. Residents live in private or shared apartments and benefit from communal dining, social activities, and transportation services. The focus is on maintaining independence while providing necessary support.

Memory Care Facilities: These specialized units or standalone facilities cater specifically to individuals with Alzheimer's disease or other forms of dementia. They offer 24-hour supervised care, structured activities, and specialized staff trained to manage the unique challenges associated with memory loss. These facilities are designed to provide a safe and secure environment with features to prevent wandering and reduce confusion.

Nursing Homes: Also known as skilled nursing facilities, nursing homes provide the highest level of care, including comprehensive medical and personal care. They are intended for individuals with serious health conditions or disabilities who require continuous medical supervision and assistance with daily activities. Nursing homes have medical professionals on staff, including nurses and doctors, and provide rehabilitation services, long-term care, and end-of-life care.

In summary, assisted living facilities offer support for daily activities with a focus on independence, memory care facilities specialize in dementia care with a safe and structured environment, and nursing homes provide intensive medical and personal care for those with significant health needs.

Recognizing When It's Time for Memory Care

Making the decision to consider memory care for a loved one is an emotional journey, filled with mixed feelings. It's like realizing that, despite your best efforts, a different set of tools is needed to provide the care your loved one truly deserves. Recognizing when it's time to make this transition is crucial. You might notice signs such as increased wandering behaviors posing safety risks or health care needs that have intensified beyond what can be managed at home. Another indicator might be the emotional strain and physical exhaustion you're experiencing as a caregiver, which can impact the level of care you're able to provide, no matter your dedication.

For a fantastic video full of tips and tidbits of great information on this topic, take a look and listen to this interview between Dr. Natali Edmonds and the co-founder of Stone Lodge Memory Care Center, Mary Jo Johnson Gibbons, here: [How and when to move someone with dementia to a nursing home](#)

Finding the Right Memory Care Facility

Choosing the right memory care facility is like finding a new home for your loved one—a place where they will not only receive the care they need but also thrive. Start with a checklist that includes essentials like the level of medical care, staff-to-resident ratio, and security measures. But don't stop there. Visit the facilities to get a feel for the environment. Are residents engaged in activities? Does the staff seem attentive and compassionate? Are the rooms and common areas clean and welcoming? Ask about daily routines and how care is tailored for residents with different stages of dementia. Inquire about how medical emergencies are handled. This information helps you visualize what daily life would be like for your loved one.

During one of my deep dives into the world of dementia care, I discovered an outstanding memory care facility that truly stands out: Bella Groves in Texas, just north of San Antonio. The co-founder and CEO, James Lee, launched this facility drawing from his extensive experience as a caregiver and various roles in senior living management. His approach to dementia care is nothing short of revolutionary, positioning the facility as a vital partner in your caregiving journey. I highly recommend watching his enlightening interview with Dr. Natali Edmonds, which I found incredibly informative. You can view it here: The Care Facility That's Transforming Dementia Care.

While Bella Groves will not be accessible to everyone reading this or exploring their website, the insights from this interview set a high standard for dementia care. **It helps equip you with the knowledge to critically evaluate any facility you consider, ensuring you ask the right questions and make informed decisions that best support your loved one with dementia**. This is a game-changer in understanding what exemplary care should look like, and I hope it inspires and empowers you as much as it did me.

Preparing for the Transition

Preparing for the move to a memory care facility involves both practical and emotional steps. Involve your loved one in the decision-making process as much as their condition allows. Discuss the move openly (as long as their mental capacity allows it; otherwise, please watch this video to get some tips on what to tell them), focusing on the positives like specialized care and new social opportunities.

On the practical side, start organizing their belongings early. Choose items from home that will make their new space feel familiar and comforting, such as favorite photos, a beloved quilt, or a familiar piece of furniture. These personal touches can significantly ease the transition. (This video, Dementia Nursing Home Transition, provides additional tips that might be very helpful as well.)

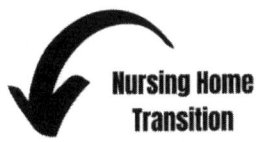

Adjusting to the New Normal

The adjustment period after the move can be challenging for both you and your loved one. Your role shifts from primary caregiver to advocate and visitor, a change that can bring feelings of guilt or relief. During this time, maintain regular visits and stay involved in their care. Communicate frequently with the staff to stay updated on their adjustment and health status. Participate in care planning meetings and continue to advocate for their needs and preferences. Engage with the facility's community by attending events or support groups. This involvement fosters a sense of belonging for both you and your loved one, smoothing the transition and reinforcing that you are still a vital part of their life.

Ensuring Quality Care

Navigating the transition to memory care is a significant step. By carefully assessing when it's needed, choosing the right facility, preparing thoroughly for the move, and actively participating in the adjustment period, you ensure that your loved one continues to receive the best possible care in a setting designed to enhance their quality of life. And if you're a fan of ratings and reviews for things like I am, you might want to check out this link to U.S. Nursing Home Ratings & Info.

However, a word of caution from someone in the industry: These ratings are only used for those facilities that accept Medicare/Medicaid, and they are not always accurate when it comes to how the staff will treat or care for your loved one. These facilities have passed inspections, and the applicable boxes were checked for the Centers for Medicare & Medicaid Services to give them such ratings. Please do **not** decide on a facility based solely on this rating chart, but I do believe it can be a helpful tool as a factor for your decision.

Navigating Healthcare Advocacy for Your Loved One

Stepping into the role of a medical advocate for your loved one is like becoming a diplomat in a high-stakes international assembly. Your mission? To ensure that your loved one's needs and preferences aren't just acknowledged but prioritized. This role is crucial, especially in the context of dementia, where patients often struggle to communicate their discomfort, pain, or even their basic needs. You are their voice, and understanding what this advocacy entails is your first step toward making a significant impact on their care. (Here's a great article from Alzheimer's News Today that will help you to understand just how important your role as an advocate is for someone with dementia.)

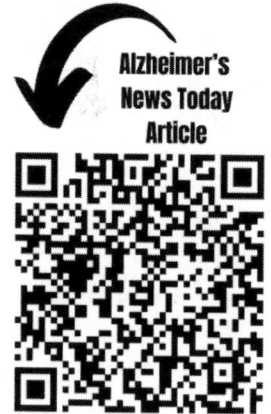

Becoming the Voice: Advocacy in Medical Settings

Effective advocacy starts with a deep understanding of the healthcare environment your loved one is wading through. This means getting to grips with treatment protocols, decision-making processes, and patient rights. Every patient has the right to respectful treatment, confidentiality, and full disclosure about their health status and available treatments. Knowing these rights empowers you to hold healthcare providers accountable, ensuring your loved one receives the quality care they deserve. Your knowledge is their shield against neglect.

Handling the paperwork and understanding the rights of your loved one during care transitions can be quite a headache. Ever thought about what to do if a hospital or care facility mixes up the paperwork during a transfer? Or how to handle the situation if you're suddenly told that your loved one's "Medicare days are up, and they need to leave tomorrow."? Do you know whether cameras are allowed in your loved one's room? Are you familiar with the differences between regulated and unregulated facilities? Or the best way to set up a written care plan for your LOWD?

Experts in elder law can be invaluable in these scenarios. The Life Care Planning Law Firms Association offers access to attorneys who not only specialize in elder law, some of them are hyper-focused on dementia care and can provide guidance on these issues. I learned about this resource from Dr. Natali Edmonds' interview with Bob Mannor from the Mannor Law Group in Michigan. His insights are useful no matter where you are. (Watch the interview here: Elder Law Advice: Advocating for Your Loved One with Dementia!)

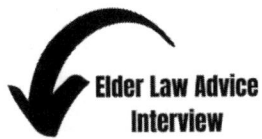

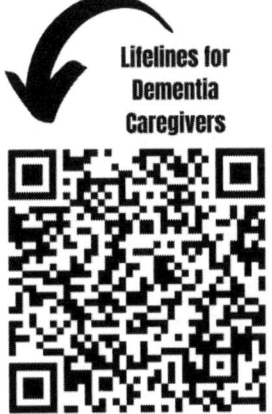

If you haven't downloaded it yet, I've included all the important links and QR codes that Dr. Edmonds provided from this very informative meeting for you (and much more) in my Lifelines for Dementia Caregivers handout—I'm afraid there just simply isn't enough room on this page to add all the QR codes for those of you reading this in print.

Mastering Medical Diplomacy for Your Loved One's Care

To navigate the healthcare system effectively, you'll need to become fluent in medical terminology and insurance intricacies. Think of it as learning a new language to unlock the best care options for your loved one. Understanding your LOWD's insurance plan can help you avoid unexpected costs and advocate for necessary treatments. If an insurance claim is denied, knowing the appeal process means you can confidently challenge these decisions. Mastering this language is key to securing the best possible care. I've spent countless hours on the phone with our insurance company learning all I can. I encourage you to do the same. *Pro tip: Don't pay **any charge** from a provider until you've confirmed with your insurance company it's legit.*

The Caregiver's Guide to Effective Medical Advocacy

At the heart of advocacy lies effective communication. It's not just about talking; it's about engaging in meaningful dialogues with healthcare professionals. Approach each conversation as a crucial negotiation—prepare your points and ask questions without hesitation. Simplify complex medical terms when necessary—"Can you explain that in simpler terms?"—to ensure you fully understand and can make informed decisions. Your goal is always clear: advancing your loved one's treatment and well-being.

Empowering Your Role: Due Diligence in Dementia Care

Sometimes, getting a second opinion is essential to explore all treatment options, especially for major medical decisions. Seeking another expert's view doesn't mean you distrust the current medical team; it's about ensuring thorough care—like getting multiple estimates before a big home improvement project. This due diligence confirms that the chosen treatment path is the best fit for your loved one's unique needs.

Knowledge is Power: Strengthening Your Advocacy Skills

Empowering yourself as a caregiver involves boosting your advocacy confidence. Educate yourself about dementia, join caregiver support networks, and attend relevant workshops and seminars. Knowledge is power—it enhances your effectiveness as an advocate. Also, recognize the emotional and psychological challenges of caregiving. Prioritizing your mental well-being helps you stay composed and assertive in demanding medical settings.

I'd like to end this chapter with some words from former First Lady of the United States, Rosalynn Carter, who said, "There are only four kinds of people in the world—those who have been caregivers, those who are currently caregivers, those who will be caregivers, and those who will need caregivers." Some of us fall into more than one of those categories, and it is vital that we are able to advocate for ourselves and anyone in our care.

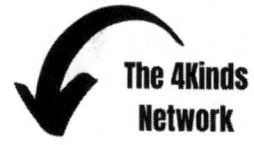

If you'd like to take your advocacy experience(s) even further, one suggestion I have is to check out the Rosalynn Carter Institute for Caregivers and learn about _The 4Kinds Network_: "a community of current and former caregivers from all backgrounds advocating for structural change to our current systems of care and supporting each other along the way. Whether you're seeking to connect with a compassionate community or to amplify your voice for change, we're here to embrace you on your caregiving journey." (4Kinds – _Rosalynn Carter Institute_, n.d.)

As we turn the page to our next chapter, we'll plunge into the depths of an issue frequently swept under the caregiving rug—self-care. You see, being a caregiver isn't just about caring for your loved one; it's equally about caring for yourself. Remember, you're the beacon lighting up their path. But to shine brightly, you must first ensure your own flame is well-tended. Taking care of yourself isn't selfish; it's pivotal. It's the unsung lesson every caregiver needs to learn, master, and practice like a sacred ritual.

Chapter 8: The Caregiver's Caretaker

"In the realm of caregiving, remember to be your own hero first. For within the cultivation of our own well-being, we find the strength to light the way for others."
–S.R. Hatton

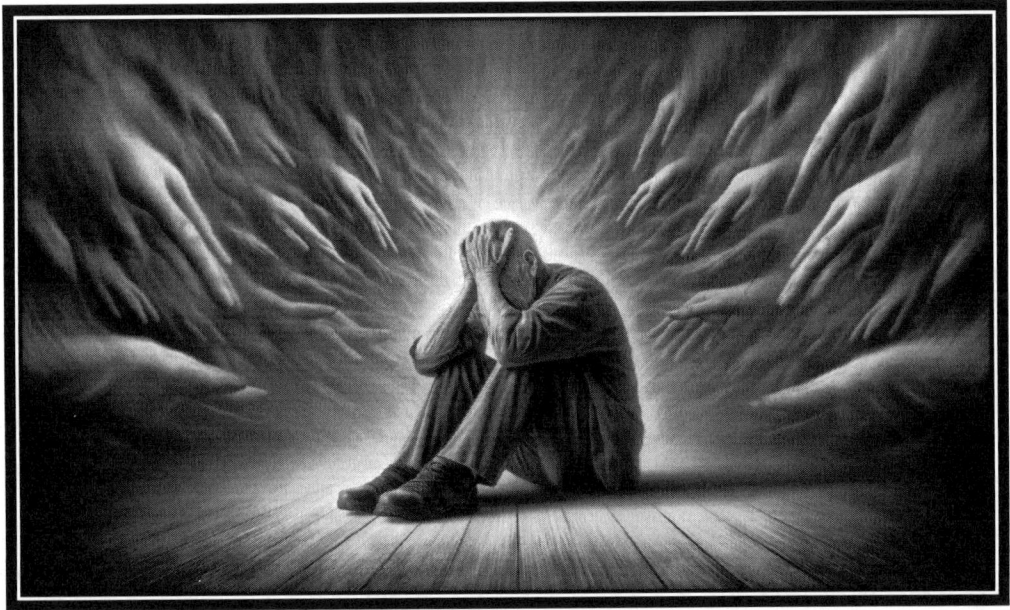

Dementia can be a formidable adversary, causing distress not only to those diagnosed but also to their loved ones. Providing compassionate support and maintaining a sense of independence is crucial, but have you been able to fully grasp what this experience is, no doubt, **doing to you and your health**?

The Invisible Second Patient—You

Caring for a loved one with dementia feels like you're in an endless maze, where each turn brings new challenges. You see glimmers of who they once were, hidden in a face that barely recognizes you. Their eyes silently plead for help when words fail them. This journey is deeply personal, tethered directly to your heart. Stress will ebb and flow, tears will flood your days, and frustration will brew storms within. Burnout might seem inevitable, but self-neglect doesn't have to be your fate.

Around 48% of caregivers who assist older adults are tending to someone with Alzheimer's or another type of dementia (Alzheimer's Association, 2024).

This caregiving role, while rewarding, comes with a unique set of challenges due to the distinct behaviors associated with dementia (Samuels, 2023):

Intense Care Requirements: Dementia caregivers often provide what's termed "high-intensity care," dealing with more complex behavioral issues and managing more activities of daily living (ADLs) than those caring for older adults without dementia. This means their caregiving duties are not only more frequent but also more demanding. *Example: Managing the full spectrum of personal care from dressing to feeding, often compounded by the need to handle outbursts or wandering tendencies.*

Physical and Emotional Toll: The strain on dementia caregivers is significantly high, manifesting both physically and emotionally. Many report health problems, increased stress, and symptoms of burnout. Social isolation and financial strain are also common as caregiving demands escalate. *In other words: Feeling continuously exhausted and isolated, while also dealing with financial pressures from reduced work hours or medical expenses.*

Prolonged Duration: Caregiving for someone with dementia typically extends over a longer period, with the median duration being around five years. This is substantially longer than caregiving for other conditions associated with aging.

Constant Supervision: Individuals with dementia often require ongoing supervision. They may not express gratitude due to cognitive impairments and are more prone to depression. *Think of it like this: Needing to be vigilant at all times to prevent accidents or manage sudden mood swings, without much acknowledgment or appreciation from the care recipient.*

Reciprocal Health Risks: The well-being of a dementia caregiver can directly impact the person they care for. Negative caregiving experiences can lead to increased depression and anxiety in both the caregiver and the recipient. Those who feel trapped or unprepared in their caregiving role often experience greater mental health challenges. *Basically: A caregiver's stress and frustration can exacerbate the care recipient's behavioral issues, creating a cycle of worsening emotional health for both.*

Additional Dementia Caregiver Challenges:

Dementia Caregiver Stress: The progression of dementia in a loved one can lead to increased caregiver stress, especially as personality changes and behaviors like aggression or wandering become more

pronounced. *Example: Feeling like you are caring for a stranger, which can be emotionally disorienting and highly stressful.*
Depression: Providing intensive care for extended periods often results in caregiver depression, worsened by the deteriorating condition of the loved one. *Basically: The realization that no matter how well you take care of them, they won't get better.*
Loneliness: The intense demands of caregiving can lead to social isolation, especially if the caregiver has limited support or respite options.
Impact on Personal Relationships: The strain of dementia caregiving can adversely affect personal relationships, such as marriage, especially where one spouse is the caregiver.

"**As long as they are clean, fed, and comfortable**, you've done your job for the moment and should take some much-needed time for yourself."—Anonymous Quora contributor

Remember, while caregiving is a tremendous task, you are more than just a caregiver. You're a human being with your own needs, aspirations, and joys. Don't forget to live your life while providing care for another.

Course Correction: Overcoming & Preventing Caregiving Mistakes

While I realize that good intentions are lighting the way on your caregiving journey, there will always be some missteps. But I urge you to learn how to stumble gracefully—mistakes are just detours to wisdom. Learn, adjust, and grow. Focus on solutions, celebrate victories, and remember that you're not dealing with a child. Here, from the Dementia Downunder Support Group (*Caring Mistakes*, n.d.), are common pitfalls and their fixes.

Common Caregiving Mistakes & the Most Common Solutions

1. **Being Disagreeable**
   - **To Do**: Embrace their world like a tourist in a strange land—full of curiosity and compassion.
   - **NOT to Do**: Resist their reality like it's a bad movie you can't turn off.

2. **Sweating the Small Stuff**
   - **To Do**: Let go and let live. If they want to put the milk in the pantry, just roll with it.
   - **NOT to Do**: Stress over minor mishaps like they're epic disasters.

The Caregiver's Caretaker | 107

3. **Arguing with Them**
   - **To Do**: Take the blame for everything. Does it really matter in the grand scheme of things?
   - **NOT to Do**: Kickstart a verbal armageddon.

4. **Correcting Constantly**
   - **To Do**: Live in their reality. If they call a cat a dog, just pet the "dog."
   - **NOT to Do**: Correct them like a strict schoolteacher grading a paper.

5. **Making Too Much Noise**
   - **To Do**: Create a Zen haven. Think spa day with soothing tunes.
   - **NOT to Do**: Turn the house into a rock concert, especially at mealtime.

6. **Ignoring Them at Mealtimes**
   - **To Do**: Focus on them like they're the only person in the room.
   - **NOT to Do**: Socialize with everyone else while they fade into the background.

7. **Speaking Too Loudly**
   - **To Do**: Keep it calm and clear—think gentle librarian voice.
   - **NOT to Do**: Shout like you're at a football game.

8. **Discussing Them in Public or with Others in the Room**
   - **To Do**: Show respect. Talk about them as if they're listening, because they are.
   - **NOT to Do**: Gossip about them like they're not there.

9. **Disregarding Their Feelings**
   - **To Do**: Validate their emotions like a good therapist.
   - **NOT to Do**: Act like their feelings are as invisible as a ghost.

10. **Taking Their Insults Personally**
    - **To Do**: Brush it off like water off a duck's back.
    - **NOT to Do**: React like you're in a personal vendetta.

11. **Lacking Humor**
    - **To Do**: Laugh often. Turn mishaps into shared giggles.
    - **NOT to Do**: Be as serious as a tax audit.

12. **Losing Your Patience**
    - **To Do**: Patience is key—apply it liberally like sunscreen. Take a deep breath and count to 5 before reacting.
    - **NOT to Do**: Snap like a twig under pressure.

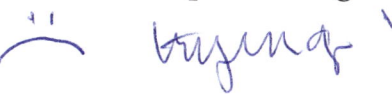

13. Ignoring Their Interests
- **To Do**: Engage them in their favorite activities like a personal cheerleader.
- **NOT to Do**: Let their hobbies collect dust like forgotten relics.

14. Resisting Adaptation
- **To Do**: Go with the flow like a river.
- **NOT to Do**: Fight the current like a stubborn rock.

15. The Choice Conundrum
- **To Do:** Roll out the red carpet of options. Whether it's choosing what to wear or deciding between tea and coffee, let your loved one take the director's seat sometimes.
- **NOT to Do:** Don't play dictator. Denying choices is like telling someone they can only watch reruns of the worst TV show ever.

16. Believing They are Misunderstanding on Purpose
- **To Do:** Keep calm and carry on with compassion. Understand that misunderstandings aren't a plot against your sanity; they're just part of the journey.
- **NOT to Do:** Don't accuse them of being sneaky with their forgetfulness. It's not a Sherlock Holmes mystery; they genuinely need your patience.

17. Moving Them Without Explaining Why
- **To Do:** Announce your actions like a gentle sportscaster. A simple touch and a soft explanation can turn a routine move into a reassuring action.
- **NOT to Do:** Don't move them like you're rearranging furniture. No one likes to be shuffled around without a heads-up.

18. Shoveling Food into Their Mouth at Mealtime
- **To Do:** Turn mealtime into a slow dance. Pay attention to their pace and encourage every bite with patience.
- **NOT to Do:** Avoid shoveling food like you're loading coal into a furnace. It's a meal, not a race.

19. Fashion Police
- **To Do:** Style them (almost) like they're hitting the red carpet. Matching socks and neatly arranged outfits can make anyone feel like a star.
- **NOT to Do:** Don't dress them in a fashion mishap. Clashing patterns might be in for runways, but let's keep their dignity intact.

20. **Strengths Spotlight**
    - **To Do:** Focus on what they can do, not what they can't. Tailor activities to their abilities and celebrate every small win.
    - **NOT to Do:** Don't set them up for failure. It's not a game show; avoid putting them in losing situations.

21. **Anger Management**
    - **To Do:** Stay as cool as a cucumber. Mistakes happen, greet them with a smile instead of a scowl.
    - **NOT to Do:** Don't turn into the Hulk every time something goes awry. They're not doing it on purpose.

22. **The 'Remember' Trap**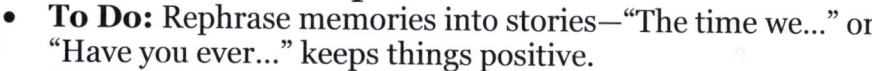
    - **To Do:** Rephrase memories into stories—"The time we…" or "Have you ever…" keeps things positive.
    - **NOT to Do:** Don't challenge their memory. Asking them to remember is like asking a fish to climb a tree.

23. **Showing Your Frustration**
    - **To Do:** Master the art of Zen. Slow down, stay calm, and let them take their time.
    - **NOT to Do:** Don't rush them. They're not in boot camp; respect their pace.

24. **Individuality Matters**
    - **To Do:** Treat them as the unique individuals they are. Customize your approach to match their preferences and stage of dementia.
    - **NOT to Do:** Don't lump their needs into a one-size-fits-all plan. They're people, not production models.

25. **Not Introducing Yourself**
    - **To Do:** Introduce yourself with a warm smile and eye contact each time you meet. A name badge can also help jog their memory.
    - **NOT to Do:** Don't assume they remember you from day to day. It's not a sitcom where everyone knows your name.

26. **Silence is Golden**
    - **To Do:** Keep it down when they're engrossed in their favorite show. A quiet environment helps them focus and enjoy.
    - **NOT to Do:** Don't crank up your noise level. If the TV is their concert, you don't need to be the opening act.

27. Repeat After Me
- **To Do:** Embrace the repeats with grace. If they tell the same story, listen like it's an encore of their greatest hit.
- **NOT to Do:** Avoid saying, "You already told me that." It's not a conversation competition; let them express themselves.

28. Your Tired Tales
- **To Do:** Keep your fatigue to yourself or share it with friends, not with the person you're caring for.
- **NOT to Do:** Don't make them feel like a burden by complaining about your tiredness. It's not a sympathy contest.

29. Changing Taste Buds
- **To Do:** Embrace their new culinary preferences with gusto! Experiment with flavors like a mad scientist in the kitchen.
- **NOT to Do:** Don't start a food fight over their newfound dislike for peas. Arguing about taste is like debating colors with a blind artist.

30. Leaving the House Without Spare Clothes
- **To Do:** Pack like you're a scout leader on a high-risk adventure—spare clothes, snacks, the works.
- **NOT to Do:** Don't leave the house unprepared. Forgetting spare clothes is like going on a road trip without gas.

31. Blaming Everything on Dementia
- **To Do:** Play detective first. Rule out pain, side effects, and other culprits before blaming dementia.
- **NOT to Do:** Don't assume every mishap is a symptom. Dementia isn't the universal scapegoat.

32. Inclusion in Daily Tasks
- **To Do:** Get them involved. Adjust tasks to their reality and make them feel needed.
- **NOT to Do:** Don't sideline them. Excluding them from daily chores is like telling Picasso he can't paint.

33. Medication Mania
- **To Do:** Stick to the script—literally. Follow medical advice to the letter.
- **NOT to Do:** Don't overmedicate them just to catch a break. Using meds as a pause button is like using duct tape for a leaky faucet.

34. **Caregiver Self-Care**
    - **To Do:** Put on your own oxygen mask first. Take breaks, stay healthy, and keep your energy up.
    - **NOT to Do:** Don't burn the candle at both ends. Ignoring your own needs is like trying to drive on flat tires.

35. **Talking Over Them**
    - **To Do:** Let them speak. Patience is your best ally in understanding their thoughts.
    - **NOT to Do:** Don't bulldoze the conversation. Talking over them is as rude as texting at a concert.

36. **Living in the Moment**
    - **To Do:** Tune into their reality. If they're back in the '60s, groove with them.
    - **NOT to Do:** Don't drag them into your timeline. Forcing them to live in the present is like asking a penguin to fly.

37. **Family Events Inclusion**
    - **To Do:** Make them part of the festivities. Their presence can enrich events.
    - **NOT to Do:** Don't exclude them. Missing out on family gatherings is like being benched at your own game.

38. **Memory Lane**
    - **To Do:** Use photos and stories to spark conversations and jog memories.
    - **NOT to Do:** Don't let their past collect dust. Forgetting to reminisce with them is like skipping the best parts of a movie.

39. **Providing Comfort**
    - **To Do:** Offer reassurance often. A touch, a kind word, and a warm tone can work wonders.
    - **NOT to Do:** Don't leave them feeling insecure. Ignoring their need for reassurance is like turning off the lights during a scary movie.

40. **TV Time**
    - **To Do:** Keep TV watching diverse and engaging. Mix in some comedies with fun documentaries.
    - **NOT to Do:** Don't use the TV as a constant babysitter. Having them watch TV all day long is also a no-no—they need some exercise and social interaction, too!

41. **Purposeful Activities**
    - **To Do:** Plan activities that have meaning and engage them on multiple levels.
    - **NOT to Do:** Don't fill their schedule with fluff. Activities without purpose are as exciting as watching paint dry.

42. **Alone Time**
    - **To Do:** Ensure they have some personal space to relax and be with their thoughts.
    - **NOT to Do:** Don't crowd them. Everyone needs a break, even from loved ones.

43. **Non-Verbal Cues**
    - **To Do:** Be observant. Recognize and respond to their physical cues.
    - **NOT to Do:** Don't ignore their signals. Overlooking a restroom request is like missing an important phone call, only messier.

44. **Respectful Conversations**
    - **To Do:** Include them in discussions about them. Speak **with** them, not **about** them.
    - **NOT to Do:** Don't talk as if they're not there. Discussing their condition in their presence without involving them is as tactful as gossiping loudly in a quiet room.

45. **Appropriate TV Content**
    - **To Do:** Choose TV channels thoughtfully. Keep content light and uplifting where possible.
    - **NOT to Do:** Don't expose them to unsettling news. It's like forcing them to live in a storm cloud.

46. **Activity Flexibility**
    - **To Do:** Have backup plans for group activities. Be ready to switch gears if the mood shifts.
    - **NOT to Do:** Don't stubbornly stick to a failing plan. Continuing with an unliked activity is like reading a bad book to the end.

47. **Inclusive Activities**
    - **To Do:** Adapt group activities so everyone can participate. Find creative ways to include all stages of dementia.
    - **NOT to Do:** Don't exclude based on ability. Leaving someone out because of their dementia stage is like not inviting someone to a party because they can't dance.

48. **Attentive Caregiving**
    - **To Do:** Treat each person with the care and respect you'd give a close family member.
    - **NOT to Do:** Don't slack in your caregiving duties. Performing tasks half-heartedly is like cooking a meal without tasting it.

49. **Respecting Modesty**
    - **To Do:** Act like a modesty superhero. Use a hand towel for cover-ups during care, ensuring privacy isn't just a courtesy—it's a guarantee.
    - **NOT to Do:** Don't treat them like an open book. Imagine how awkward it would be if someone narrated your every move in the bathroom!

50. **Rushing Through Daily/Weekly Tasks**
    - **To Do:** Turn daily tasks into a Zen ritual. Wash their hair with the care of a spa technician and find joy in the small moments.
    - **NOT to Do:** Don't rush like you're late for a flight. Treating care tasks like a race only leads to skinned knees and bruised egos.

51. **Outdoor Access**
    - **To Do:** Be their sunshine manager. Regularly escort them outdoors for a healthy dose of vitamin D and fresh air.
    - **NOT to Do:** Don't keep them cooped up like a winter hermit. Denying access to nature is like saying no to a free mood booster.

52. **Gentle and Caring Approach**
    - **To Do:** Communicate with the tenderness of a favorite kindergarten teacher. Make eye contact and speak softly, explaining your actions carefully.
    - **NOT to Do:** Don't be forceful or uncaring. Acting like a cold, unfeeling robot can make them feel more like a task than a person.

53. **Personal Terms of Endearment**
    - **To Do:** Use their name like it's a golden key that unlocks more meaningful interactions.
    - **NOT to Do:** Don't sprinkle generic sweet-nothings like "Sweetheart" or "Dear" as if they're seasoning. It's impersonal and bland.

54. **Tone of Voice**
    - **To Do:** Speak naturally, respecting their adulthood. Your tone should convey respect, not condescension.
    - **NOT to Do:** Don't sing your words in a high-pitched voice. You're talking to an adult, not serenading a baby.

55. **Using Lifting Equipment Safely**
    - **To Do:** Handle all equipment like you're a pro technician. Ensure straps are placed comfortably and safely (especially in their nether region).
    - **NOT to Do:** Don't be careless with setup. Incorrect strap placement can lead to discomfort or even injuries, making it feel like an amateur wrestling match gone wrong.

56. **Dignity in Delicate Situations**
    - **To Do:** Act like a dignity ninja. Use discretion during potentially embarrassing moments, using whatever you can to shield them from other eyes, and handle accidents with utmost respect.
    - **NOT to Do:** Don't make a scene or highlight mishaps. Commenting on odors or a mess is as tactful as a bull in a china shop.

57. **Encouraging Independence**
    - **To Do:** Support their abilities by encouraging them to participate in their care and daily activities.
    - **NOT to Do:** Don't do everything for them. Treating them like a life-size doll removes their dignity and is actually counterproductive.

58. **Night Comfort**
    - **To Do:** Think of them like a sleeping beauty. Ensure they are comfortable all night with appropriate bedding for the season.
    - **NOT to Do:** Don't neglect their nighttime needs. Imagine lying in a cold bed with all your blankets on the floor—and you're unable to get them. How would you feel?

59. **Supervised Outdoor Time**
    - **To Do:** Keep a watchful eye during outdoor activities to ensure safety and comfort.
    - **NOT to Do:** Don't ever leave them unattended. Forgetting about someone in the sun is like leaving cookies in the oven—bound to become burnt.

60. **Proper Posture Care**
    - **To Do:** Pay attention to how they sit or lie down. Adjust their position to prevent discomfort.
    - **NOT to Do:** Don't ignore their body alignment. Staying in the same position all day long can lead to pain, making you the villain in their story.

61. **Respectful Room Entry**
    - **To Do:** Always knock and announce your presence. It's simply a courtesy, like ringing a doorbell.
    - **NOT to Do:** Don't barge in. Bursting into their room unannounced is as rude as skipping the queue at a coffee shop.

62. **Acknowledge Non-Verbal Communication**
    - **To Do:** Pay close attention to all forms of communication, ensuring they feel seen and heard.
    - **NOT to Do:** Don't overlook those who aren't verbally expressive. Ignoring their attempts at communication is like muting the TV during the best part of the show.

Unchecked Stress: The Silent Saboteur in Caregiving

Caregiving is a labor of love, but it must never blind us to our own well-being. You, the caregiver, matter as much as the loved one you're caring for. The specter of burnout constantly looms over caregivers who neglect their own self-care. Astonishingly, some even spiral into states of anxiety and depression more severe than those they are caring for—rendering them the silent victims of this journey. Sofia Amirpoor, a seasoned caregiver, frequently shares pearls of wisdom in her video chats. She has witnessed the toll this journey exacts on caregivers—tear-streaked faces, sleepless nights, and an overwhelming sense of stress. In the direst of instances, caregivers have suffered heart attacks and strokes. One particularly tragic event saw a caregiver's stress culminate in a fatal house fire, claiming her life and her mother's. According to Amirpoor, these harrowing stories underscore the importance of self-care as a survival tool for caregivers (Amirpoor, 2020).

Unchecked stress is a silent infiltrator, waging a slow, destructive war on your body, mind, and spirit. This is why it's pivotal for you, the caregiver, to remain vigilant against the dangers of sustained, unattended stress. And remember, you're not alone in this journey. Reach out, connect, share—lean on support groups, friends, and family. If geographical barriers stand in your way, let the digital world bring the support to you.

As a caregiver, your days will oscillate between moments of triumph and trials. Embrace this reality, and arm yourself with the knowledge to better navigate the landscape of care. Every dawn brings with it a fresh opportunity to learn and grow, not just as a caregiver but also as an individual with dreams and aspirations.

"Toxic caregiver stress" is a gradual, insidious process. It isn't an overnight transformation. Instead, it accumulates, day after day, week after week, till it becomes a silent, looming behemoth. Imagine your stress as a pressure cooker, each day's troubles adding more heat, inching it closer to its boiling point. **It's crucial to remember that the stress you're attempting to evade doesn't simply dissipate into thin air. It finds a home within you, building up until it results in a state of extreme burnout**. This isn't merely an abstract concept—it's a reality that demands your utmost attention.

Shaping Your Stress: From Chronic Burden to Healthy Catalyst

In this chapter, we will unravel the art of transforming the cumbersome chains of chronic stress into a galvanizing force, one that we'll refer to as 'healthy stress.' By making self-care a non-negotiable part of your routine, you bolster your resilience to the rigorous demands of caregiving. The strength of your fortress against chronic stress is directly proportional to how well-prepared you are. Healthy stress can be a productive motivator, pushing us beyond our comfort zones without leaving scars, while chronic stress, even when it appears innocuous, can gradually erode our well-being.

This might sound a little counterintuitive, but some of the most effective advice calls for caregivers to cultivate a measured degree of selfishness. After all, to be the best caregiver you can be, you must prevent yourself from sliding into a role where you also need caregiving! Now, let's look into the distinction between chronic and healthy stress and learn how the right mindset and a willingness to embrace positivity can morph chronic stress into a constructive companion.

Remember, healthy stress isn't just beneficial; it's achievable, and it holds the key to better care for yourself and your loved one. As you strive to banish chronic stress from your life and embrace healthier alternatives, you're embarking on a journey of renewal. By consciously making choices that enhance your well-being, you're opening doors to a healthier, more balanced life, steering clear of the damaging aftershocks from uncontrolled stress.

Every day presents an opportunity for you to bolster your physical and mental health. It all begins with a shift in perception, from viewing stressors as harbingers of doom to seeing them as challenges you can conquer with positivity and resilience.

Consequences of Chronic Stress	**Consequences of Healthy Stress**
👎 Chronic stress endangers your health.	👍 Also known as "eustress," good stress invigorates your life.
Wreaks havoc on your body and mind.	Adds a positive thrill to your existence.
Meddles with your immune system.	Eustress steers clear of negative emotions.
Hinders digestion and reproduction.	Choosing activities and setting goals that excite you create eustress.
Triggers anxiety and depression.	Creating a self-care routine to support your caregiving goals can boost self-esteem.
Leads to weight gain.	Eustress motivates you to view challenges positively.
Causes muscle tension and pain.	Caregiving under eustress benefits you and your loved one.
Can induce heart disease, stroke, and high blood pressure.	Embracing your self-care routine transforms stress.
Impairs memory and concentration.	Goal setting under eustress makes caregiving more manageable.
Disrupts healthy sleeping patterns.	Balancing caregiving with personal life under eustress enhances rest and rejuvenation.

In this pursuit, remember that not all negative stress can be transformed into the healthier variant. Nevertheless, we can certainly fine-tune our responses to stress, preventing negative emotions from taking the driver's seat. Here's how you can kick-start this transformation:

1. **Actively harness your resources** to counter challenges, consistently evaluating what you need to better meet your own and your loved one's needs.
2. **Seek ways to enhance your support system**. Join caregiver forums, indulge in regular exercise to ward off stress, or consult a therapist to improve your coping skills.

3. **Celebrate your strengths and invest in self-improvement.** By understanding your capabilities and focusing on nurturing them, you'll gain confidence to tackle any obstacle or setback that comes your way.
4. **Prioritize planning.** A well-thought-out plan reduces stress and arms you with the tools to manage challenges effectively. By setting meaningful goals and taking proactive steps to achieve them, you're not just preparing for the days ahead; you're crafting a purpose-filled journey for yourself and the one you care for (Scott, 2023).
5. **Practice positive thinking whenever possible.** Start by using a concept called "Notice-Shift-Rewire," which is further explained here in this article: _The Neuroscience of Breaking Out of Negative Thinking (and How to Do It in Under 30 Seconds)_.

What Is Caregiver Burnout?

Burnout among caregivers is a formidable reality that affects those battling the demanding tides of balancing care for their loved one with dementia and their personal lives. Often, caregivers, in their noble mission to provide the best care, sideline their own well-being, pinning unrealistic hopes on their abilities and those of their LOWD. This pressure cooker situation has led some caregivers to the brink of nerve-shattering breakdowns—a testament to the severity of the emotional strain that dementia caregiving can induce. Some caregivers even feel entrapped, as if they had no choice but to take on this role, further pushing them into a vortex of stress, lack of preparation, and an unbalanced life.

But listen closely, you do not have to walk this path.

Your journey can be different. By prioritizing self-care, enhancing your knowledge, managing your life effectively, and finding equilibrium between your own needs and those of your LOWD, you can prevent your story from becoming another tale of a burned-out, self-pitying caregiver. Embrace caregiving as a rewarding experience rather than a jail sentence. Your liberation lies in the trinity of action, accountability, and a positive attitude.

Here, let's delve into the real-life experiences of two caregivers, Dana and Leah, shared on an online support forum for caregivers:

Dana laments, "I loathe caregiving. The guilt weighs heavily on me, but the truth remains. I've lost my life to it. Yes, I seize fleeting moments for myself when the hired aide is present, but it barely eases the constant pressure that envelops me. Caregiving feels like a colossal responsibility that's ended my life. Despite the antidepressants, they don't alleviate my emotional pain; the side effects are simply horrific. I dread the void my mom's departure will leave, but for now, my life feels finished. I'm searching for solace but finding none." — Anonymous Quora Contributor

Meanwhile, Leah shares, "Two years ago, I left my job to care for my mom, who started forgetting me. Ever since, my home feels like a fortress I rarely leave. Hiring a sitter for a few hours a week during the first year was more of a financial drain and a source of depression than a relief. As I pen this, the echo of my mom's distress as she attempts to rise from her bed resonates in my ears." —Anonymous Quora Contributor

Understanding these experiences is critical, as it could be the key to you navigating this journey differently.

Here are the signs of burnout to be on the lookout for (Cleveland Clinic, 2019):

- Social isolation
- Loss of personal interests and hygiene
- Feeling depressed, irritable, and hopeless
- Changes in appetite which can result in weight fluctuations
- Disrupted sleeping patterns
- Falling ill more often
- Destructive feelings and behavior
- Bad moods, experiencing intense anger
- Physical exhaustion
- Emotional tiredness or numbness

Burnout Quiz

Are you dancing on the edge of caregiver burnout? It's an abyss that can sneak up on you, masked by what seems like everyday stress. The AARP offers a valuable tool—a caregiver burnout quiz. If your score veers toward the high end, it's a red flag. It's time to take action, not just for your well-being, but for your ability to continue providing the care your loved one depends on. Healing starts with acknowledging your struggle and taking steps to restore your mental and physical strength.

Your score rating is on a scale from one to seven. Take the quiz and see where you stand—it's the first step towards understanding and managing your caregiver burnout. (If you prefer a printable copy that you can download and write in your scores, click on this quiz sheet or scan the QR code to the right.)

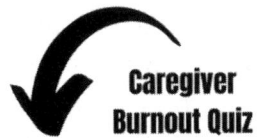

(1 Point) This never happens.
(2 Points) Maybe once.
(3 Points) It is rare.
(4 Points) Sometimes.
(5 Points) Yes, often.
(6 Points) It is very usual.
(7 Points) Always.

In caring for a loved one, how often do you have the following experiences:

Quiz Questions

1. Feelings of resentment come up while caring for your LOWD.
2. You feel trapped in a hopeless situation.
3. You're tired more often and don't get enough sleep at night.
4. You feel weary.
5. You feel helpless.
6. You tend to overeat a lot, or you have a poor appetite.
7. You are physically exhausted.
8. Feelings of disillusionment overwhelm you.
9. Everything feels hopeless and dull.
10. You are drained of feelings.
11. You're unhappy.
12. You're anxious.
13. You're stressed all the time.
14. You're depressed.
15. You feel rejected and useless.

Take a moment and think: How are you really feeling? If your score falls below 60, breathe a sigh of relief—you're maintaining a balance between your caregiving responsibilities and personal well-being. However, if your score climbs to 90 or above, it's a glaring sign that you're deep in the trenches of caregiver burnout. It's time for an intervention (*Caregiver Quiz*, n.d.).

Here are some restorative actions you can embark on to relieve stress and reclaim control:

1. **Prioritize your health**: Rethink your dietary habits, steering away from the pitfalls of substance abuse, alcohol, or smoking. Resist the siren song of sugary binges, instead embrace wholesome snacking

like fruits and vegetables. Prioritize a full night's sleep, but if nighttime rest eludes you, a daytime nap can recharge your batteries. Experience the healing power of nature, let your feet wander, and allow exercise to become a regular part of your routine. Embrace activities that uplift you—it's a great way to boost those 'happy hormones,' the endorphins, which will help combat stress and foster positivity.

2. **Keep the lines of communication open**: Isolation is a breeding ground for stress. Stay connected with family and friends and engage in their lives. Stimulating and meaningful conversations can create a healthy escape from your daily caregiving routine, bringing the vibrant world back into your life. Another option is to join the amazing Facebook groups that are especially for caregivers of a loved one with dementia. These groups have thousands of members who are doing exactly what you are doing: caring for their LOWD. Just enter the keyword "Dementia" into their 'search' function, review the rules of the group, and then ask to join. It only takes a moment, and then you'll be privy to very valuable information. You can also ask any questions you have and get answers and advice that you might not ever have found in your inner circle of friends and family.

3. **Permit yourself a break**: You're allowed to pause. Explore community services in your area and consider hiring extra help. This way, you can find time to engage in activities that interest you. Remember, your loved one, in their healthy state, would want you to enjoy life, too. It's about finding that equilibrium between their needs and yours. Use the eldercare locator to find your local Area Agency on Aging (or other resources located in my *Lifelines for Dementia Caregivers* handout). Then give them a call and find out what resources are available to you. Something called "respite care" may be an option—and according to caregivers, it can be worth its weight in gold, and then some.

Eldercare Locator

4. **Plan a getaway**: Why not envision a dream holiday? Utilize health agencies or a nursing home for your loved one's care during your absence. Or perhaps delegate care responsibilities to other family members. As long as your loved one is well-cared for, you deserve a respite—an adventure just for you.

122 | Dealing with Dementia for Caregivers

5. **Nurture a positive mindset**: If resentment is brewing, it's crucial to address it. Identify negative patterns in your life and understand that you may need help breaking these cycles. Try to focus on the positives and seek solutions to improve your emotional state. Sometimes, gaining a fresh perspective means taking a step back, especially during heightened emotions. Don't hesitate to seek therapy if you're stuck in a negative spiral. Remember, reaching out is not a sign of weakness, but a courageous step towards breaking free from the clutches of burnout before it escalates into a crisis.

Are you on the quest for assistance in the United States? Your answer could be Visiting Angels. This organization offers a broad spectrum of services, including home care, respite care, dementia care, palliative care, and even end-of-life care. All you need to do is input your zip code, and you'll find the closest facility (Visiting Angels, n.d.).

If you're navigating through this journey in the UK, consider reaching out to Admiral Nurses. These are your knights in shining armor, specialized dementia nurses who provide transformative support for families battling the waves of all forms of dementia (Dementia UK, 2023).

Remember, the right help can be a game-changer. It's essential to explore these avenues, as they can provide invaluable support during this challenging journey. Don't walk this path alone. The help is out there, and it's just a zip code or phone call away.

Real-World Tips & Tricks to Deal with Caregiver Burnout

Being Reasonable, Rational, and Logical Will Just Get You into Trouble. Rational explanations don't work well for those with dementia; straightforward and simple communication is more effective.

People with Dementia Do Not Need to Be Grounded in Reality. Rather than reminding someone with dementia of painful truths, redirect their attention by discussing their memories or asking about their experiences.

You Will Never Be the Perfect Caregiver: Accept that you cannot be the perfect caregiver; only do your best and endeavor to improve.

Honesty Can Lead to Distress for Dementia Sufferers: It is not always the best policy. Engage in therapeutic lying for both of you to have better days. Don't stress yourself out by always telling them the truth.

Don't Make Agreements with Them to Get Them to Do Things: They will soon forget, and this will create stress for you. Accept that they will forget things more easily than usual.

Be In Charge: You need to educate their doctors and others about their likes and dislikes, their behavior, and if they are showing signs of increased agitation, so make a note of things. ***Pro tip: Keep a daily journal.***

Accept Help: Accept that it is impossible for you to do everything yourself. You will need help, so get it when you recognize that help is needed.

Take Things One Day at a Time: Every day will be different, so do not judge progress based on previous days. Go with the flow and be prepared for new challenges.

Tell Them Things and Don't Ask Them: For example, don't ask them what they would like for dinner; tell them when it is time for dinner.

It's Never Personal: Remember that when they are agitated, in a rage, or being difficult, it is not personal. You, as the caregiver, are no longer just responding to your LOWD; you are responding to the disease (*Ten Real-Life Strategies for Dementia Caregiving - Family Caregiver Alliance*, 2022).

In traversing the endless streams of caregiving advice on Facebook Groups dedicated to those caring for loved ones with dementia, I stumbled upon a remarkable tip, one that is as valuable as it is bittersweet. **Look to those who have traversed the same path you're on, and whose journey has reached its end due to the passing of their loved ones.** It may seem melancholic, but these individuals, laden with hard-earned wisdom and surplus time, can be your respite, your helping hand.

Imagine this: Someone who has walked in your shoes, stepping in to assist you for a few hours, allowing you that precious time to rejuvenate and nurture yourself. To run errands without worry, to indulge in a long, relaxing bath, to take a tranquil drive where you can immerse yourself in thought, or simply catch up on the restorative sleep that seems so elusive.

Reaching out is the first step—make an online post detailing your needs, your available time slots, and your location. You might be pleasantly surprised by the number of willing and capable people who are ready to lend a hand.

Here's a sneak peek into other valuable tips I've discovered that could make a world of difference to your caregiving journey:

"While caregiving is often a labor of love, tending to someone with dementia can go beyond merely draining

your energy—it can leave you so dry it's debilitating, and in some cases, it can even lead to severe health issues.

Now, what could possibly be the 'single best thing' to counteract this debilitating process? In my view, it would be to share the load with a professional—a nurse or someone with medical training. This gives you the breathing space you need to maintain your own health and well-being—to shower, rest, recharge, and occasionally step outside to reconnect with the world beyond the confines of your caregiving environment.

Another worthwhile consideration would be a night nurse, a guardian angel of sorts. A good night's sleep can make all the difference—it's often the pivot between perseverance and total exhaustion.

Even if you can only afford to bring in help for just a few days a week, it makes a significant impact on your own well-being.

But what if the 'best thing' isn't an option? Well, there's still plenty that others can do to lighten your load. Help with housekeeping, laundry, sorting mail, paying bills, maintaining the home, or even running errands like picking up prescriptions—every little bit of assistance contributes to easing your burden.

Consider another option—someone could take charge of meal preparations, ensuring your refrigerator is perpetually stocked with wholesome, easy-to-consume meals. Or they could pop by for a visit, bearing a prepared meal as a welcome treat.

Let's not forget, the caregiver's emotional well-being also requires nurturing. A comforting friend who listens, offers a shoulder to cry on, or provides a change of scenery—such as a leisurely walk, a cup of coffee, or even a movie. Naturally, this break would be dependent on someone else being present to care for the person with dementia.

Being a caregiver often feels like you're suspended in a timeless space while life outside continues to ebb and flow. Children grow up, friends undergo life changes like marriages, divorces, or career advancements. So, be that lifeline—the tether that connects the caregiver to the outside world. You just might be the buoy that preserves her sanity, or even saves her life." —Anonymous Quora Contributor

In those moments when you feel you've come to the end of your rope, when your LOWD is exhibiting aggressive and challenging (maybe even dangerous) behavior, refusing to bathe, hydrate, or take their necessary medications, know that you're not alone. Many have been in your shoes and have found ways to turn the tide. Here are some potentially life-changing tips that other caregivers have discovered and generously shared, tailored to situations just like yours:

"At hospice, we had a little packet of compounded meds in lotion form. It was used specifically for agitation and her type of behavior. It consisted of Ativan, Benadryl, Haldol, and Reglan (for nausea). Ask your doctor to write a script of it in the lowest doses and send it to a compounding pharmacy if he agrees. IT WORKS WONDERS…slip it on the back of her neck when she [is out of control]. I am not practicing medicine, nor am I prescribing. Just passing along a trade secret. Good luck."—Facebook Group member

****

"Yes, call 911 and say she's threatening self-harm and has hit you, you need help. They SHOULD send an ambulance and take her to the ER for an evaluation. They usually admit them for [a] 72-hr hold and try to figure out if they need their meds adjusted or if they need a psych evaluation. Push for the psych evaluation and with luck they will admit her for 14 days. If you do not accompany her to the ER, that's your choice, give the EMTs the phone numbers of ALL the other family members, then turn your phone off and get some sleep. Please don't let her come back to your home, take care of you and let the professionals take care of her."—Facebook Group member

"To add to everyone:
Please keep a journal.
Take pictures and videos (use your phone to video).
This way, you have proof [in order to get medications for the aggression]. It's a Horrible situation."
—Facebook Group member

****

"Many assisted living facilities (and even MC [Memory Care] places) offer short-term respite care—loved ones to stay with them—so caregivers can get breaks. It would buy

you time to find placement options in peace."—Facebook Group member

****

"I don't know about all states, but would imagine other states have something similar. My mom never prepared for this time in her life. In AZ, we have Arizona Long Term care services (ALTCS). We got her qualified with the dementia diagnosis, and she went into assisted living. State pays for everything except her SS amount which is paid by me to the assisted living facility. It was a God send as I couldn't manage her and my full-time job. I would imagine each state would have something similar?" —Facebook Group member

****

"I would suggest you to contact the local social worker from department of aging—if that's not possible, contact an elder care attorney who can advise you of the options you have (sometimes the first consultation is free); if that does not work, contact local church or a not for profit foundation. They will be able to provide a slate of options for the area you are in; in terms of options, in my mind, you have 3; (1) Hire private caregivers for few hours to help you gain your sanity back;(2) look for a short term respite care to check mom in followed by some hours from private caregiver 3 to 4 times a week;(3) get her situated in an assisted living; Again, sitting afar, it's difficult to suggest which option is best for you!" —Facebook Group member

****

"I have a caregiver that comes to my home Mon-Friday from 9 to 2:30 we got the help through her insurance through Medicare and Medicaid we called customer service and ask for a Care Coordinator that came and did an assessment called NFLOC and she was approved for 27 hours a week and 250 hours a year for respite care." — Facebook Group member

As we tread gently into our next chapter, we're faced with an emotional reality inherent to the journey with dementia—the farewell. It's a challenging, inevitable crossroads filled with profound emotions and essential preparations. Guided by deep empathy, my hope is to get through this heartfelt chapter as supportively as possible, easing the path toward understanding and readiness for this profoundly personal experience.

Chapter 9: Handling the Inevitable with Grace

"When life's final act draws near, may the star of the show bow out surrounded only by the peace and love in your silent ovation." –S.R. Hatton

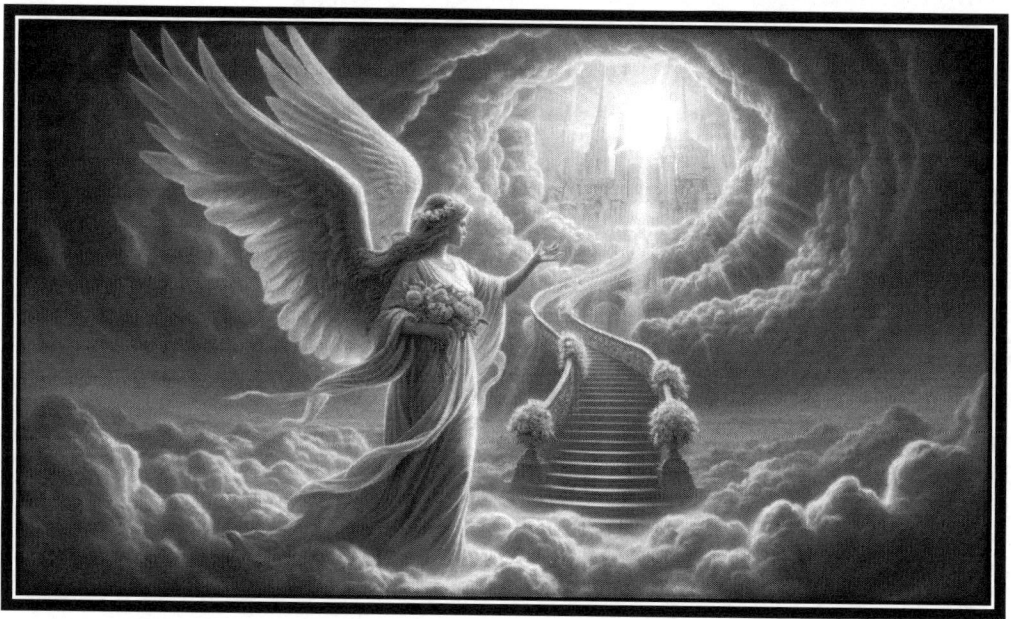

I Hate, I Hate, I Hate!

For five days straight, all my mom said on her deathbed was, "I hate. I hate. I hate." Every "I hate" that she uttered broke my heart. I wanted to believe that she was trying to communicate with me in some metaphysical way that did not translate into the literal meaning of those words. Still, it stung me, and the only thing available to do was to console her as best as I could. In my mind, I wondered what she meant. Maybe, I thought, she was telling me to water her plants three times a day. All I had to go on in her last hours were those words, "I hate, I hate, I hate." There was nothing I could do to console her or to find out more. She was dying from dementia, the hateful sickness that made her hate. I tried to decode those words. I was grasping at straws, trying to figure it out, trying to enlighten myself and lessen the burden of those words.

Maybe she was telling me to eat Hi-fiber, I thought, or she was telling me to tie my shoelaces. Sometimes, she said, "Eat Hi" or "Ha tie" (as a joke to tie my shoelaces). However, eventually, I realized there was no hidden message in those words, "I hate." I desperately didn't want those words to be her last words, but that's all she said on her deathbed. Of course, I tried to console her by telling her that everything was going to be okay. "You are loved. You are loved. You are loved. Everything is going to be okay."

My mom hated doctors. She also hated people telling her what to do and fussing all over her. I held her hand. It was clenched tightly into a fist. So, I placed my hands on top of hers. She started fading away. I knew she was leaving me. For three days, I sat with her witnessing her facing death with those dreaded words, "I hate. I hate. I hate." Perhaps she was negotiating with death. There must have been some tough negotiations going on between her and death. Finally, after a couple of days, she was moved to the hospice. It was almost time to say my final goodbyes. Moving her to the hospice was better. There was no fussing. She hated that.

The atmosphere was more peaceful. I looked like I hadn't taken a shower since the '90s. Mom's hand stayed in a clenched fist. When I gently opened her fist to massage the palms of her hands, she warmed up. It was just mother and son. Two souls saying, "Goodbye. Until we meet again." We sat there. She smiled at me. I told her it was going to be okay. "You are loved." She whispered back to me, "Okay." Those were her last words. My mom passed away a day later. I imagined that she was in God's arms now, safe, free, and at peace (Roedel, 2022).

The Expected Visitor

You will never be fully prepared for the death of your loved one. You will know that the time will come soon when their condition worsens. There is no amount of words one can write about being prepared for that moment because it will not amount to much. And I don't mean that in the way it sounds—the grief starts when they are diagnosed, and it continues in cycles: even when you feel resentful while caring for them, you will still be haunted by the grief of losing them to dementia. They don't call it the 'long good-bye' for nothing.

As the disease progresses, it takes more of them each time until you are left with only their body—their soul is locked up somewhere in there, unable to fully communicate with you. They may smile through their eyes and look at you, feeling comforted by your presence. You will never know what they are thinking or feeling in their last moments. It will hurt more. That is why having soulful conversations while they are still in the early stages is important. You might be left with, "I hate. I hate. I hate." or the memory of another hallucination. However, know this—as long as their soul is with you, they are with you. The words will fail them. It doesn't mean anything anymore.

As you begin caring for them now, in the early days, as I am assuming you are still in the early days of your journey as a caregiver—seeking answers to anything and everything—see it as a blessing, and remember these words, "I hate, I hate, I hate." You don't know what words will greet you in their last days or last hour. You might get an "okay." You might get nothing at all. As you begin to care for them, remember that it will get worse. You will face their last days with them. You will feel the burden of this grief that accompanies dementia for many days, on and off, while they are still with you. **Begin your journey as a caregiver with the end in mind**.

One day you will be saying goodbye to them, and it may come sooner than you think. Make their in-between comfortable, special, and filled with activities. Let them have their way. Do what you can to ease the days they have left and your days with them, and be kind to them. It is not going to be an easy journey. It can be a blessed one, and you will grasp at straws of hope. You will wish this never happened to them. You will want them back before they are gone. It will not change anything. Don't expect perfection in your journey. It will get much worse one day. You will not be prepared for the final loss. However, you can heal and have peace, too, knowing their ordeal has ended. Peace will find them.

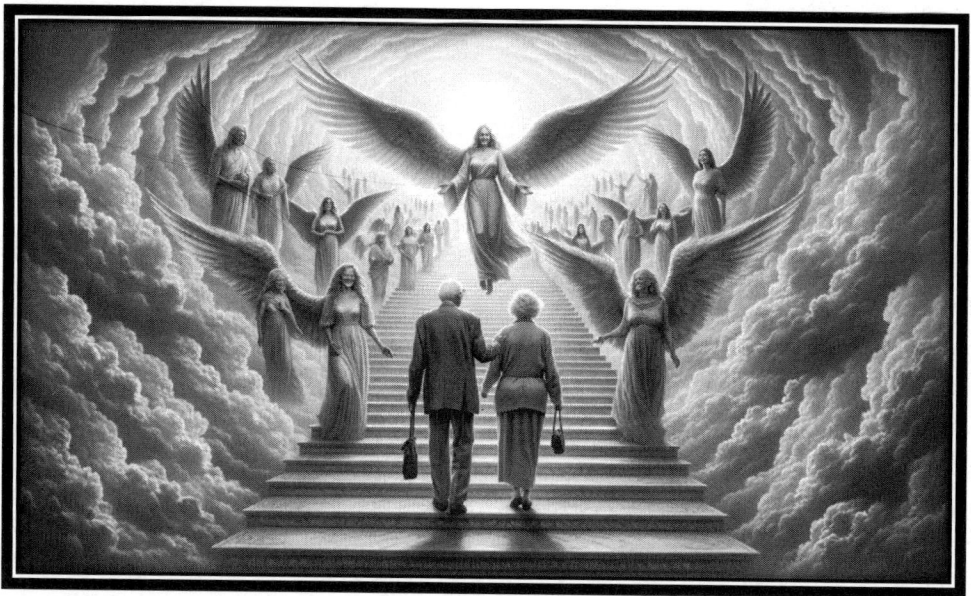

Reaching the End of the Road with Dementia

You may ask, how can I prepare for their death? Will there be signs, a warning? Or will it be thrust upon me out of the blue? There are signs when it's time to start saying goodbye to your loved one. Unless they have a sudden stroke or heart attack, there will be clear signs for you. Keep in mind that nothing is guaranteed in life. However, the end signs of life with dementia are clear enough to recognize.

Regardless of what type of associated neurological diseases they suffer from that cause dementia, the end days of your LOWD will be marked by specific late-stage dementia symptoms. To be prepared, always have their legal affairs in order, and **be ready every day for anything**.

Here are the signs of late-stage dementia, also called end-stage dementia, which should be a clear enough indication that your LOWD is in the grip of its last stages—when brain damage is permanent.

1. They need help with all basic functions.
2. They cannot speak anymore.
3. They are incapable of even lifting up their head.
4. They will not be able to walk, talk, or do anything by themselves.
5. They may get other illnesses like pneumonia, which can also cause death.
6. They eat less and experience difficulty swallowing food.
7. Bowel and bladder incontinence are common in the late stages.
8. They lose consciousness.
9. They become more agitated and very restless.
10. Their speech is limited to one or two words.
11. Their hands and feet are cold.
12. You'll hear chesty, heavy breathing

When your loved one is in the final stages of life, it would be wise to get the help of a healthcare professional. They are trained to know how to assist a dying dementia patient. Their care for your LOWD will be invaluable. Healthcare professionals can make it more comfortable for your loved one when they are in their final stages by easing their pain and administering medication to ease their discomfort. If your loved one cannot swallow food or medication, they will be able to inject them accordingly with medication (*How to Know When a Person With Dementia Is Nearing the End of Their Life*, 2021).

Real-World Advice on Facing Death

The very best advice I found as to how to handle the moment of their death is this: **Nothing.** There is nothing to do when they die. There's no need to rush around to call the nurse to ease their pain, suffering, or inability to comprehend things. There is no schedule to follow, a bed to be made for them, or reassurances you need to give them anymore. It's all over after they die.

Just sit there and be silent to take in the magnitude of the moment that has occurred.

"Don't panic. They are at peace now. There's no need to frantically phone people. Not just yet. Be silent and cherish your journey in that one moment that they fade away. Take a moment to connect silently with their traveling soul. As morbid as it might sound, it is a sacred moment when a soul transitions to the next life. I believe in an afterlife. They are traveling. They've been set free from their suffering. Honor that freedom. Honor the end of their suffering. Feel your grief at losing them. Yet feel their newfound freedom begin somewhere else. The heavens will embrace them now. When death arrives, the veil between the two worlds is parted. An angel comes to get them, to take them away on a new journey—to take them back home, where all is well. There is no sickness there. No dementia. They will remember you.

Be still when this happens. Take it in. Do you feel a presence? Do you feel their peace? Allow yourself to feel what comes up for you as they transition. If you are religious or spiritual, say a prayer out loud. Let them hear you if they can, as you will feel their essence in the last moments. As they slip away, you will be moved by the parting and the soul leaving its body. Wish them love. Wish them a blessed journey to the afterlife. Death will shock you. Yet you must prepare your words for them for the final hour." —Quora contributor

Thank You, I Love You

"What will you say to them? For that, you can prepare. Think about it. Say it out loud even while they're alive. Say those words that say everything. It's only five words. Say it many times over while they are with you. You can thank them softly during your time together. Say, 'Thank you. I love you.' What will you do when they leave you? Will you wonder if you were a great caregiver or mother, daughter, son, sister, brother, husband, or wife?

When their soul departs, spend at least ten minutes doing nothing. Breathe deeply. Close your eyes. Say your final words. What will complete that moment for you? If you can't think of any words, just remember these, 'Thank you. I love you.' Move slowly. Call one person at a time. Take your time to get the words out of your mouth. Don't miss the moment, though—it is a gift to be in the presence of a soul that has just left its body. Part of them is still there.

You must honor them by being still. Cry softly if you want. Be with them. Be gentle. Move softly. Respectfully. Thankfully. In gratitude for their contribution to your life. Be grateful that you were there to receive the blessings of being there, regardless of how bumpy and imperfect those days may have been. Remember them. Their smiles. Their frowns. Their rage. It was all of them inside." —Quora contributor

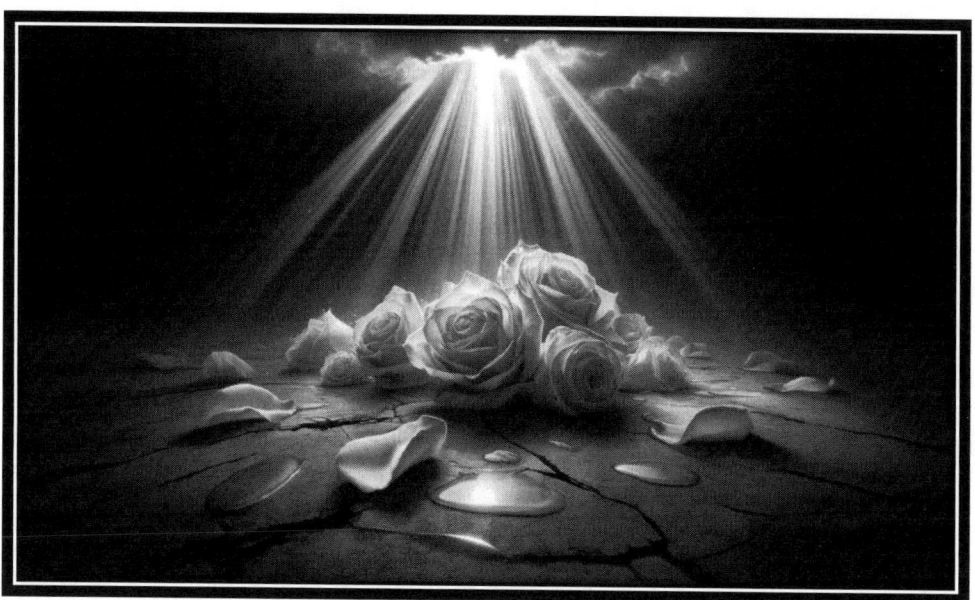

Conclusion

As we draw close to the end of this guide, I want to emphasize something that may seem simple, yet it's profound: Love is all that truly matters. If you speak with anyone who has lost a loved one to dementia, they'll tell you about the invaluable power of love through the caregiving journey. The hours spent worrying about whether you're doing enough, coupled with the struggles with guilt, helplessness, and resentment, might feel overwhelming. Yet, it is love that will carry you and your loved one through these turbulent times.

In the throes of caring for someone with dementia, it's crucial to remember that love isn't just a feeling—it's a practice. It involves learning new ways to connect, ensuring their safety, and adapting your home to meet their changing needs. It's about balancing the care they need with the personal goals and dreams you continue to hold for yourself.

Yes, the threat of adverse events is real if they're not properly supported, which is why we've discussed how to create a safer environment. But more than safety, love is a catalyst for growth and validation. It helps you persevere during tough times and find fulfillment in seeing your loved one secure and appreciated in their new reality. Every effort to make them feel safe, loved, and understood is a step towards giving them peace beyond their days.

Hope for a cure is natural and understandable. It fuels our actions and decisions to seek the best treatments and stay informed about medical advances. However, it's also vital to maintain a balance—to hope without losing ourselves in it. We are caregivers, not medical professionals, but we offer our best with the tools currently available.

This book is not just a collection of tips; it's a testament to the unique value of your experiences, which have shaped the collective wisdom of many who have walked this path before us. As we continue to learn about the brain and dementia, we remain hopeful for breakthroughs that could one day reverse the course of this illness.

So, as you move forward, keep love at the forefront of everything you do. It's the most potent medicine we have. Share what you've learned here with others who might benefit, and let your experiences inspire and uplift others in the caregiving community. Remember, you're not just doing enough—you're making a profound difference.

I wish you strength, joy, and endless love in your journey ahead. You are part of a community that thrives on mutual support and collective wisdom, and your presence and contributions are deeply valued.

Epilogue

I want to take a minute here to bring your attention to something that holds some promise for those of us touched by this horrible condition. I've been keeping an eye on two brothers, Professor Lars Ittner and Dr. Arne Ittner, who are researchers at Macquarie University's Dementia Research Centre in Australia. They have made one of the most promising and thrilling breakthroughs in the fight against Alzheimer's and other dementia-related diseases.

In a jaw-dropping development, these genius siblings have found a new treatment that not only halts but reversibly sweeps away the cobwebs of memory loss in mice with advanced dementia. Their secret weapon? A naturally occurring brain enzyme known as p38gamma, which they've managed to harness to block the toxic effects that lead to memory loss. When activated through their innovative gene therapy, this enzyme acts like a memory shield, bringing the mice not just back to baseline but restoring their ability to learn—effectively turning back the clock on their cognitive decline.

The implications of this discovery are monumental, promising a future where Alzheimer's and frontotemporal dementia—diseases that devastate millions, including younger adults in their prime—could be effectively treated or even cured. Imagine a world where memory loss is no longer an inevitable slide into oblivion but a reversible glitch. That's the world the Ittner brothers are pioneering, and their results are so groundbreaking that they themselves are "really stoked" about the potential (K. Cox, 2020).

Watch this YouTube video (New hope as dementia therapy reverses memory loss) to hear about their "eureka moment." Dr. Arne Ittner is also featured in this more recent video (Investigating p38gamma's role in protecting against dementia).

Upon learning about this breakthrough, Macquarie University established Celosia Therapeutics to focus on advancing this gene therapy through clinical trials and (hopefully) gaining approval for use in human patients.

Please spread the word to anyone and everyone who might want to follow their research. This is one of the brightest beacons of hope I've seen on the horizon of dementia research—let's pray that they are able to turn the tide in our favor and reverse this cruel, mind-killing disease.

Share Your Knowledge: A Call to Guide Fellow Caregivers

"True generosity means planting trees under whose shade you do not expect to sit." —Anonymous

You've just navigated the twists and turns of *Dealing with Dementia for Caregivers*—congratulations! Now, how about one more adventure? Leaving an online review can light the path for those just stepping into their caregiving shoes.

Think of it this way: Your words could be the lighthouse guiding lost ships through a stormy night. Wouldn't you want to be that guiding light for someone else?

Here's the scoop: People often pick books based on what previous readers say, not just the blurb on the back cover. So, your mission, should you choose to accept it, involves a little keyboard wizardry on behalf of the next generation of caregivers.

Would you be willing to sprinkle some of that magic dust for someone you've never met? Here's how your review can save the day:

1. **Illuminate the Path**: Shine a light on how this book guided you through the fog. What chapters were your guiding stars?
2. **Pass the Compass**: Highlight the practical tips that steered you right. Which strategies were your North Star?
3. **Gather the Troops**: Every review adds a leaf to the family tree of caregivers, creating a canopy of collective wisdom.

Ready to cast your spell? It's as easy as holding your phone camera over the QR code to the right—It'll zip you over to the Amazon review platform where you can pour your potion of wisdom into the caregiving kettle.

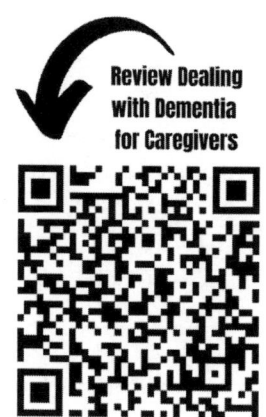

Thank you for deciding to pass on the torch. Your insights are not just words; they're the compass for future caregivers navigating their map of challenges. By sharing your experience, we continue to forge a path of empathy, aid, and shared knowledge—one review at a time.

References

4Kinds – Rosalynn Carter Institute. (n.d.). https://rosalynncarter.org/4kinds/

7 stages of Lewy Body dementia. (n.d.). MeasurAbilities, LLC. Retrieved June 8, 2024, from https://measurabilities.com/7-stages-of-lewy-body-dementia/

10 must-dos when serving as a caregiver for family, friends. (n.d.). https://www.americanbar.org/news/abanews/publications/youraba/2017/april-2017/a-10-step-legal-checklist-for-caregivers-/

10 ways to make your home dementia friendly. (n.d.). Alzheimer's Society. https://www.alzheimers.org.uk/blog/10-ways-make-your-home-dementia-friendly

ADI - Dementia statistics. (n.d.). ADI - Dementia Statistics. https://www.alzint.org/about/dementia-facts-figures/dementia-statistics/

Alex, C. (2023, April 6). *2.1 Your emotional reaction to the dementia diagnosis*. Forward With Dementia [UK]. https://www.forwardwithdementia.org/en/article/2-1-your-emotional-reaction-to-the-dementia-diagnosis-being-told-someone-close-to-you-has-dementia-brings-up-strong-emotions/

Alzheimer's Association. (2024). 2024 Alzheimer's disease facts and figures. In *Alzheimers Dement* (Vols. 20–5). https://www.alz.org/media/documents/alzheimers-facts-and-figures.pdf

Alzheimer's Society. (n.d.). Making your home dementia friendly. In *Alzheimer's Society Publication*. https://www.alzheimers.org.uk/sites/default/files/migrate/downloads/making_your_home_dementia_friendly.pdf

Amirpoor, S. (2020, May 12). *CAREGIVER BURDEN AND SEVERE CAREGIVER BURNOUT* [Video]. YouTube. https://www.youtube.com/watch?v=BiWBw-mCa0A

Andrews, L. (2023, February 16). *Bruce Willis' double diagnosis: How aphasia can lead to dementia*. Mail Online. https://www.dailymail.co.uk/health/article-11760261/Bruce-Willis-devastating-double-diagnosis-explained-aphasia-lead-dementia.html

Baldwin, E. (2020, December 17). *Let Me Go by Christina Rossetti. Poem Analysis*. https://poemanalysis.com/christina-rossetti/let-me-go/

Botek, A. M. (n.d.). *The importance of creating a daily routine for dementia patients*. AgingCare.com. https://www.agingcare.com/articles/daily-routine-for-people-with-dementia-156855.htm

Caregiver quiz. (n.d.). https://assets.aarp.org/www.aarp.org_/articles/learn/sidebars/4-quiz.htm

Caring Mistakes. (n.d.). Dementia Down Under. http://www.dementiadownunder.com/caring-mistakes/

Cherry, K. MSEd, (2022, September 27). *Hypnosis as a therapeutic tool.* Verywell Mind. https://www.verywellmind.com/what-is-hypnosis-2795921

Cleveland Clinic. (2019, January 13). *Caregiver Burnout.* Cleveland Clinic. https://my.clevelandclinic.org/health/diseases/9225-caregiver-burnout

Cobb, D. (2024, February 27). *Medicaid & Assisted Living: State by State Benefits & Eligibility.* https://www.payingforseniorcare.com/medicaid-waivers/assisted-living

Communicating with someone with dementia. (2023, February 13). NHS.uk. https://www.nhs.uk/conditions/dementia/living-with-dementia/communication/

Cox, D. (2018, September 3). Seven ways to help avoid dementia. *The Guardian.* https://www.theguardian.com/lifeandstyle/2018/sep/03/seven-ways-to-help-avoid-dementia

Cox, K. (2020, July 30). *New hope as dementia therapy reverses memory loss.* The Lighthouse. https://lighthouse.mq.edu.au/article/july-2020/New-hope-as-dementia-therapy-reverses-memory-loss

Cpmi. (2014, December 9). *A Caregiver's Story: Getting into a Dementia Patient's Head.* Brain Matters Research. https://brainmattersresearch.com/a-caregivers-story-getting-into-a-dementia-patients-head/

Creamer, J. (2018, July 30). *Dementia didn't rob me of my mom. It revealed her truest self.* America Magazine. https://www.americamagazine.org/faith/2018/07/30/dementia-didnt-rob-me-my-mom-it-revealed-her-truest-self

Daily care plan. (n.d.). Alzheimer's Disease and Dementia. https://www.alz.org/help-support/caregiving/daily-care/daily-care-plan

Dementech. (2022, December 21). *What are the 7 stages of vascular dementia? | Dementech Neurosciences.* Dementech Neurosciences. https://dementech.com/2022/06/28/what-are-the-7-stages-of-vascular-dementia/

Dementech. (2023, July 18). *What are the 7 Stages of Frontotemporal Dementia? | Dementech Neurosciences.* Dementech Neurosciences.

https://dementech.com/2022/11/10/what-are-the-7-stages-of-frontotemporal-dementia/

Dementia Care: Keeping loved ones safe and happy at home. (2024, February 8). Johns Hopkins Medicine. https://www.hopkinsmedicine.org/health/wellness-and-prevention/safe-and-happy-at-home

Dementia UK. (2023, June 21). *What is an Admiral Nurse? | Dementia UK | Specialist dementia nurses.* https://www.dementiauk.org/get-support/what-is-an-admiral-nurse/

Dementia UK. (2024, April 17). *Creating a life story for a person with dementia - Dementia UK.* https://www.dementiauk.org/information-and-support/living-with-dementia/creating-a-life-story/

Diagnosis. (2018, August 1). Stanford Health Care. https://stanfordhealthcare.org/medical-conditions/brain-and-nerves/dementia/diagnosis.html

Duff, S., & Nightingale, D. (2007). Enhancing quality of life through hypnosis. In *Alzheimer's Care Today* (Vols. 8–4, pp. 321–331). https://hypnosishealthinfo.com/wp-content/uploads/2012/12/Alternative-Approaches-to-Supporting-Individuals-With-Dementia.pdf

Five things we learned from Reagan's Alzheimer's. (2016). Right at home. https://www.rightathome.net/blog/5-things-we-learned-from-reagans-alzheimers-a

Hearing loss and the dementia connection. (2023, August 2). *Johns Hopkins Bloomberg School of Public Health.* https://publichealth.jhu.edu/2021/hearing-loss-and-the-dementia-connection

Home Safety for Families Living with Alzheimer's. (n.d.). Home Instead. https://www.homeinstead.com/care-resources/alzheimers-dementia/home-safety-considerations-families-alzheimers/

How to get a parent tested for Alzheimer's and dementia | Take care. (n.d.). https://getcarefull.com/articles/how-to-get-a-parent-tested-for-alzheimers-and-dementia

How to know when a person with dementia is nearing the end of their life. (2021, September 3). Alzheimer's Society. https://www.alzheimers.org.uk/get-support/help-dementia-care/recognising-when-someone-reaching-end-their-life

Jackson, J. L., & Mallory, R. (2009). Aggression and Violence Among Elderly Patients, a Growing Health Problem. *Journal of General Internal Medicine, 24*(10). https://doi.org/10.1007/s11606-009-1099-1

Kiger, P. (2022, July 29). *Sitting too much may be bad for your memory.* AARP. https://www.aarp.org/health/brain-health/info-2018/sitting-memory-loss-dementia

Lawrence, K. (2018, October 16). *How I coped with my mum's dementia - When They Get Older.* When They Get Older. https://whentheygetolder.co.uk/health/mental-health/understanding-dementia/how-i-coped-with-my-mums-dementia/

Learner, S. (2023). *Alzheimer's Society hopes Thatcher's death will help tackle the stigma of dementia.* Homecare. https://www.homecare.co.uk/news/article.cfm/id/1559713/alzheimers-society-hopes-thatchers-death-will-help-tackle-stigma-of-dementia

Loneliness and social isolation linked to serious health conditions. (n.d.). https://www.cdc.gov/aging/publications/features/lonely-older-adults.html

Medical Hypnosis with Roger Moore. (2023, November 27). *Hypnosis for Dementia and Alzheimer's Disease | Medical Hypnosis with Roger Moore.* Medical Hypnosis With Roger Moore | Medical Hypnosis With Roger Moore Offers Comprehensive Hypnotherapy Solutions for Weight Loss, Parkinson's, Cancer, Pain, Dementia, End-of-life, Stress and Anxiety, and Autoimmune Disease. https://hypnosishealthinfo.com/medical-hypnosis/hypnosis-dementia-alzheimers-disease/

Moore, R., Duff, Simon PhD, & Nightingale, Daniel PhD. (2007). Hypnosis for dementia. In *Alzheimer's Care Today* (Vols. 8–8, Issue 4, pp. 321–331). Palm Desert Hypnosis. https://hypnosishealthinfo.com/wp-content/uploads/2019/11/Hypnosis-for-Dementia-article-Se-Ot.pdf

Morris, S. Y. (2023, July 27). *Dementia and incontinence: is there a link?* Healthline. https://www.healthline.com/health/dementia/incontinence-care

Morrow, A., RN. (2023, August 26). *8 Ways to manage sundowning (Late-Day Confusion).* Verywell Health. https://www.verywellhealth.com/sundowing-recognize-and-manage-sundowning-1132472

Palm Desert Hypnosis. (2020, July 7). *MEDICAL HYPNOSIS - Palm Desert Hypnosis.* https://palmdeserthypnosis.com/medical-hypnosis/

Penn Medicine. (2020, December 31). *The 7 Stages of Alzheimer's Disease.* Penn Medicine. Www.pennmedicine.org. https://www.pennmedicine.org/updates/blogs/neuroscience-blog/2019/november/stages-of-alzheimers

Reduce your risk of dementia. (n.d.). Alzheimer's Society. https://www.alzheimers.org.uk/about-dementia/managing-the-risk-of-dementia/reduce-your-risk-of-dementia

Roedel, J. (2022). *Upon Departure*. Independently Published. https://www.amazon.com/Upon-Departure-John-Roedel/dp/B09X3WYJ9R

Samuels, C. (2023, December 11). *6 major health risks for dementia caregivers*. https://www.aplaceformom.com/caregiver-resources/articles/health-risks-for-dementia-caregivers

Scott, E., PhD. (2023, September 27). *The benefits of good stress*. Verywell Mind. https://www.verywellmind.com/what-kind-of-stress-is-good-for-you-3145055

Seladi-Schulman, J., PhD. (2022, June 30). *Understanding the link between dementia and depression*. Healthline. https://www.healthline.com/health/dementia/dementia-and-depression#is-depression-a-symptom

Social Care Institute for Excellence (SCIE). (2014, September 24). *Living with dementia* [Video]. YouTube. https://www.youtube.com/watch?v=loksPQ7Q8tM

Tariot, P. (2019, June 19). *Facing Fear, Facing Alzheimer's: Why Early Dementia Diagnosis Is a Must*. BeingPatient.com. https://www.beingpatient.com/early-signs-dementia-alzheimers-diagnosis-test/

Ten Real-Life Strategies for Dementia Caregiving. (n.d.). Family Caregiver Alliance. https://www.caregiver.org/resource/ten-real-life-strategies-dementia-caregiving/

The middle stage of dementia. (2021, February 24). Alzheimer's Society. https://www.alzheimers.org.uk/about-dementia/symptoms-and-diagnosis/how-dementia-progresses/middle-stage-dementia

USA Today, P. R. U. (2020, September 2). "His brain was so compromised": Robin Williams' widow describes his "devastating" final days in new doc. *USA TODAY*. https://www.usatoday.com/story/entertainment/movies/2020/09/01/robin-williams-widow-robins-wish-documentary-lewy-body-dementia/5677962002/

Vieira, Dr. K. (2015, November 16). *Stages of Mixed Dementia*. BrainTest. https://braintest.com/stages-of-mixed-dementia/

Visiting Angels. (n.d.). *Senior Home Care | Visiting Angels*. https://www.visitingangels.com/

Wandering. (n.d.). Alzheimer's Disease and Dementia. https://www.alz.org/help-support/caregiving/stages-behaviors/deambulacion

What is dementia? | CDC. (n.d.). https://www.cdc.gov/aging/dementia/index.html

What is dementia? Symptoms, types, and diagnosis. (2022, December 8). National Institute on Aging. https://www.nia.nih.gov/health/alzheimers-and-dementia/what-dementia-symptoms-types-and-diagnosis#signs

Wilkes, M. (2018, June 8). *Meg and Keith's experience of dementia with Lewy bodies and Parkinson's disease dementia.* Alzheimers.org.uk. https://www.alzheimers.org.uk/blog/meg-keith-dementia-lewy-bodies-parkinsons-disease-dementia

Yatawara, C., Lee, D. R., Lim, L., Zhou, J., & Kandiah, N. (2017). Getting Lost Behavior in Patients with Mild Alzheimer's Disease: A Cognitive and Anatomical Model. *Frontiers in medicine, 4,* 201. https://doi.org/10.3389/fmed.2017.00201

Made in the USA
Monee, IL
11 December 2024